Low Back Treatment Guide

Adults & Seniors

Carson Robertson DC

Alpha Dog Marketing LLC
4955 S Alma School Rd#10
Chandler, AZ 85248
robertsonfamilychiro.com

Copyright © 2020 by Carson D. Robertson DC

All rights reserved. This book or any portion thereof may not be reproduced or used in any manner whatsoever without the express written permission of the publisher except for the use of brief quotations in a book review.
First Published August 2023 by Alpha Dog Marketing LLC
4955 S Alma School Rd#10
Chandler, AZ 85248
https://www.robertsonfamilychiro.com/

ISBN: 9798657396935

The patient pictured on the cover was unable to properly follow directions or perform any exercises or stretches, so we do not have any active exercise pictures for the cover. My dad's best skills are talking and looking for golf balls, which did not aid in this photo shoot. When you see him in the office please tell him to wear a helmet on the motorcycle, stop repeating stories, get a hearing aid, and that the Seattle Seahawks are not the best team in football. Thank you for your help.

Table of Contents

Chapter 1: Introduction	1
Chapter 2: Anatomy of the Spine	5
Chapter 3: Imaging	23
Chapter 4: Just Getting it Done	26
Chapter 5: Chronic Low Back Pain	30
Chapter 6: Treatment Philosophy	49
Chapter 7: Spinal Stabilization -Working On The System	69
Chapter 8: Common Phrases From People Who Make Bad Decisions	79
Chapter 9: Mistakes People Make	83
Chapter 10: Scapula & Mid Back	87
Chapter 11: Scapular Dyskinesis & SICK Scapula	94
Chapter 12: Healing Process	99
Chapter 13: Chiropractic Adjustments	102
Chapter 14: Conservative Therapy	109
Chapter 15: Soft Tissue Treatments	111
Chapter 16: Graston Technique	115
Chapter 17: Shockwave Therapy	119
Chapter 18: Class IV Cold Laser	122
Chapter 19: Acupuncture & Dry Needling	125
Chapter 20: Cupping	127
Chapter 21: Traction	129
Chapter 22: Spinal Decompression	130
Chapter 23: Injection Therapies	138
Chapter 25: Home Products	145
Chapter 26: Common Surgery Questions	158
Chapter 27: Low Back Exercises	166

Chapter 1: Introduction

One of my least favorite tasks is describing a three-page MRI report to a patient. The office visit comes down to 15 minutes of crushing a person's hopes and dreams for an easy fix.

A one-page MRI report means the person is in great shape, has minimal degenerative changes, or only has one area of significant concern. Two pages are common and usually mean a few mild problems, or one or two moderate problems in the spine. Three pages always means there are multiple problems throughout the lumbar spine.

A three-page report usually corresponds to years of low back pain that the person ignored. These are the individuals who have been having more frequent bouts of back pain; in other words, a few moderate and a couple severe episodes per year for multiple years in a row. The low back has been getting worse despite fewer activities.

For example, whenever a person walks or stands for longer than half an hour, his or her back tightens and becomes sore. Vacuuming and mopping are a constant source of pain. Riding in a car for longer than an hour leads to increasing soreness. Working in the yard becomes a game of Russian Roulette; will the back hurt tomorrow or not? Occasionally bending down to pick up a shoe leads to a pop and week of severe lower back pain.

Alex was a patient in his 50s who hated his job promotion that required him to travel for work once or twice a month. Each trip involved multiple plane rides, hotel beds, long customer meetings, and usually dinners with clients. The long days compounded with different beds led to significant back pain by the time he returned home. It was common for him to spend the weekend in pain, and would often require working from home a few days so he could work from bed or laying on the floor.

He had given up on riding his mountain bike and exercise was limited to walking. Any type of lifting or running would lead to back pain. He avoided any type of vacation that involved long car or plane rides, and would often schedule his vacation days after work trips so he could recover without anyone knowing how bad his back had become.

Yes, he had a three-page report. I wish the radiologist would have just led with a statement that said, "this back is FUBAR (Fouled Up Beyond All Recognition); there are too many damaged locations for you to remember tomorrow. So make it a priority to improve your core strength, flexibility, and posture; or simply have surgery and deal with spinal fusion problems in 15 years."

I said: "Your back is like a jenga set, after pulling some of the blocks. It is wobbly and unstable. The shearing has trashed most of the lumbar discs, and arthritic changes in the vertebral body and joints are creating significant narrowing for the nerve roots and spinal cord. If facet joints were tires, you would pretend you didn't see they were all bald for months and replace all four immediately."

As you can tell, I am not the warm and fuzzy person in the office. I prefer blunt facts, risk factors, options, and proper expectations. I told Alex his low back and functional abilities were going to deteriorate if he didn't do something about it and make it a priority in his life. If he wanted to use our office for pain management only, we could do that but he needed to acknowledge which direction he was heading.

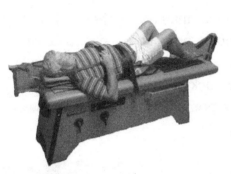

I'm not a total buzz kill. I did tell Alex a story about Nick who had a similar MRI report. Nick's wife actually brought him into the office because he had basically given up. Nick was in his 30s and was miserable. He couldn't sit, stand or walk for any significant period of time. He couldn't play with the kids without aggravating his back. The week before, he had hurt himself in the pool when one of the kids wanted to be tossed, and spent the last few days on the floor. Nick's work also required travel, which was absolutely miserable.

Nick's back was FUBAR and a jenga set: combination of multiple disc bulges and herniations with early facet and spinal degenerative changes. It was the worst MRI I had seen for someone his age.

We created a new set of exercises based on him. I previously had the basement range of motion exercises when a person couldn't handle basic movement exercises, and we needed even easier exercises. After working with Nick, I created the Bat Cave Exercise Series, for those far below the basement and are either in a James Bond villain lair or superhero hideout.

Nick dedicated himself to the home exercises and habit modifications. Each week he showed progress and was able to do more at work and home. Within two months he was playing with the kids on the floor without severe pain. He progressed through the exercise series and experienced consistent progress. His pain was improving each week, along with his quality of life.

Over the course of six months, he went weeks without back pain, and was performing exercises he had never dreamed possible. He transitioned from our office to a personal trainer with a progression of exercises.

Two years later I was running on a treadmill and saw a person performing difficult rehabilitation exercises on an exercise ball. He was working on single leg stability and squats on a BOSU with a single barbell. Very seldom does one ever see a person performing these exercises in a gym. Then I realized it was Nick. His back pain was gone and function had improved to levels beyond his imagination. He put in the hard work and deserved every pain-free day.

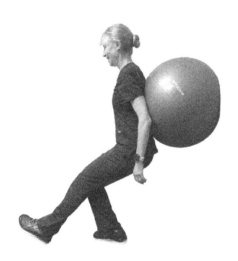

Most people do not work as hard as Nick or improve the way he did. Most motivated people follow Alex's path. They work hard and make progress for a while, then feel pretty good so they back off the exercises that created the improvement. They stop focusing on improving their sitting and standing postures. Ultimately, they experience a flare up and then recommit to the little things for a while. When work and home life get busy, they back off the exercises again, leading to another flare up after a business trip.

This book contains information on lumbar disc injuries and available treatment options. Every person is starting from a different position, but everyone can improve and enhance his or her quality of life. The activities that people avoid due to back pain are possible to resume with the right treatment plan. Few put in the work to be Nick, but I have seen many Alexs enjoy a better quality of life with these treatments.

Video: Lower Back Treatments

Everything About Life Can Be Learned in DayCare

Patients become discouraged by ups and downs during and following treatment, with cycles of improvement and aggravation. The patient thinks the pain has resolved, only to have it flare up again, often with no obvious trigger.

This cycle occurs because the musculoskeletal system is compromised. It is not a single tendon that is hurt, but rather a system-wide breakdown that has led to compromised movement patterns driven by multiple dysfunctional muscles and tendons. These changes may occur prior to the onset of pain.

Patients are often surprised when I tell them the source of their pain is not the problem. Many have concluded that years of flare ups are from a single spot or location, what else could it be? I think of my son's daycare class. Within a room full of three-year-olds, some of the kids are great, while others who are not playing well fly under the radar and avoid being noticed. Eventually members of the latter group are going to torment another kid to the point of an outburst. The kid that acts out is usually not the problem, but rather the perpetrators that are tormenting and pushing the crying child's buttons.

Once the teacher calms down the child in distress, his or her next actions determine what happens during the rest of the day. If the teacher does not address the children causing the problem, the cycle will continue throughout the entire day, making everyone's lives miserable. It would also not be surprising to find the same group of children causing problems down the road.

In the case of chronic low back injuries, soft tissues become the crying kid in daycare. In this case, muscular dysfunction and movement patterns lead to excess stress on the tissue until injury causes pain.

A therapy office can always treat what hurts to decrease pain. However, dysfunctional movement patterns will inevitably lead to reinjury.

Think of Nick's story and process in the introduction of this book. Treatment can always decrease the acute pain, but solving chronic injuries and system dysfunction requires a different process. Usually people need to be motivated and know their "why" to commit and follow through with a lifestyle and exercise improvement plan. So what is your pain causing you to miss, what is your why?

Chapter 2: Anatomy of the Spine

We ask the lower back to absorb a tremendous amount of force, strain, and stress, all while providing an exceptional range of motion. Think of all the bending, reaching, pulling, carrying, jumping, and lifting you can do because of the structure of the lower back.

To understand lower back pain treatments, it is important to review all the structures and potential pain sources.

The Spine

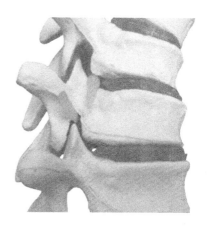

The spine was designed to be exceptionally mobile and protective at the same time. If the spine was a single bone, people would have the flexibility of a bug. Instead, the skull sits on seven cervical, twelve thoracic, and five lumbar vertebrae. The last lumbar vertebrae (5th) transfers all of the body weight to the sacrum, which then transfers the weight to two ilium through the sacroiliac joints.

Body weight is transferred between each spinal vertebrae through discs in the front and facet joints in the back. Discs and facet joints structurally support body weight and allow for movement. Facet design and structure allow for the differences in movement between the neck, upper back, and lower back.

The design of the joints between the skull and first cervical vertebrae allow for fifty percent of flexion/extension movements, or looking down to your chest and up to the sky. The structure between the first and second cervical (neck) vertebrae produces fifty percent of rotational movements, or looking over the shoulder. The direction and shape of facet joints change throughout the spine.

Vertebrae become bigger and more supportive moving from the head to tail bone, because of the increased weight load they support. Larger weight loads increase mechanical strain across joints, leading to increased risks of injury. More forces mean more injuries.

The vertebral column creates small openings for nerves to exit (neural foraminal canal) and travel through the body. The holes are behind the vertebral bodies and in front of the facet joints. Disc bulging or extruding backward can compress the nerve, creating changes in muscle strength, pain sensations, or loss of feeling. Nerve compression can also occur with facet arthrosis, which grows forward into the neural foraminal canal.

The vertebral column also creates a protective ring for the spinal cord to descend from the brain to the lower back. The spinal cord is surrounded by several protective layers and cerebrospinal fluid. Disc herniations and vertebral body bone spurs can push backward into the canal, compressing the spinal cord.

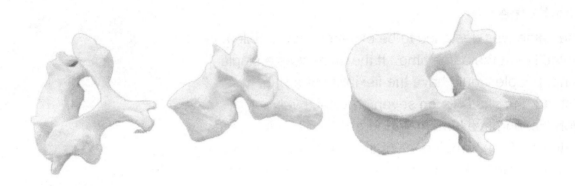

Spinal Discs

Spinal discs are located between the vertebrae. They essentially function as shock absorbers between the bones. Each disc has a thick fibrous outer layer with a fluid center. Discs help the vertebrae rotate, glide, and tip, enabling our body to move. In addition to movement, the discs also provide support. Video: Spinal Disc is like a Jelly Donut

In its shape and composition, a spinal disc is very much like a jelly donut, with the jelly in the center. If excessive pressure is applied to the donut, jelly can shoot out the back. This is similar to a spinal disc herniation, in which the fluid leaks out the back of the disc.

Unfortunately, the spinal cord and nerve roots are directly behind the spinal disc, so when excessive pressure is applied, the extruded fluid compresses either the spinal cord or nerves. Inflammation and fluid surround the herniation and further compress the nerves.

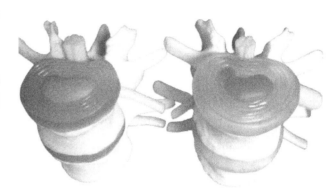

Compression of a nerve alters its function and overall health. Severe nerve compression can cause muscle weakness in the hand or foot that the nerve sends signals to. Pain, numbness, and tingling are common sensations felt by someone experiencing a disc herniation. Other people may experience a loss of skin sensitivity.

What Is Facet Arthrosis?

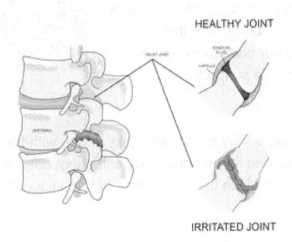

Facets are the surfaces of bone that face each other. The bone above has a column of bone that sits atop the column from the bone below. The two bones create a joint that allows for movement. There are two facet joints at each level; one on the left and the other to the right. Facet joints enable movement, but they are also weight bearing. Facet joints help transfer your body weight from above to below, along with the discs.

Disc damage results in loss of disc height and places extra strain on the facet joints. Advanced disc disease results in damage to the facet joints through wear, tear, and excessive strain.

Video: Facet Joint Sprains Are Causes of Low Back Pain

In some people with a history of disc injuries, the disc eventually becomes less painful and the facet arthrosis becomes the source of chronic pain. For this reason, disc replacement surgeries do not always relieve pain, while facet injections can relieve chronic pain.

What Does Mild, Moderate, Severe Degeneration Mean?

I refer to these terms as "a little, some, and a lot." For terms that every provider can quantify, the radiologist has to describe the changes in the standard system utilizing mild, moderate, and severe.
Standardized descriptions enable your provider to read the MRI report and explain the images to you. A

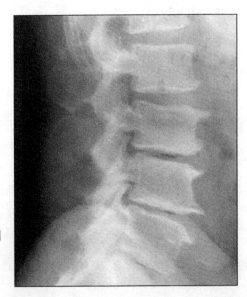

provider has likely seen a couple hundred moderate degenerative disc disease images with mild neuroforaminal narrowing, and can draw the spine from the radiologist report with pretty good accuracy (assuming your provider can draw, and I can't so my drawings are always out of scale and ugly - that's why I really like modern technology and being able to pull the images onto a computer screen for show and tell).

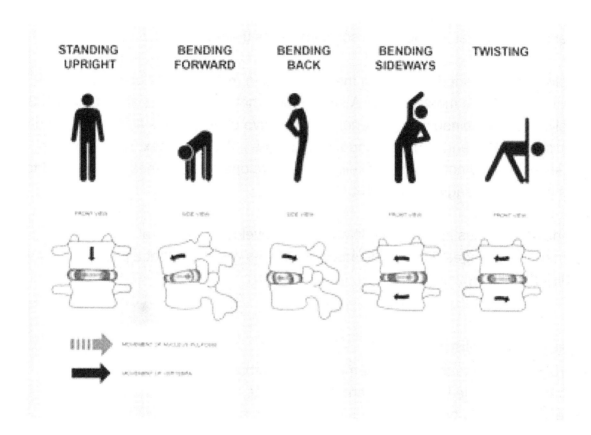

What Is Spinal Canal Stenosis?
Usually due to vertebral body arthritis or disc bulge pushing backwards into the spinal canal. A little stenosis is not always a problem as the spinal canal has extra room; however, moderate and severe degenerative changes can compress the spinal cord. The bigger the disc herniation and the more levels involved, the greater the problem.

What Is a Neural Foraminal Canal?
The nerve leaves the spine in between two vertebrae by holes created by the vertebral bodies, pedicles, and facet joints of two adjoining vertebrae. Usually the holes have plenty of extra space for the nerve. Facet arthrosis and disc herniations can cause narrowing of the neural foraminal canal and result in nerve compression.

What Is Retrolisthesis?

This occurs when the vertebral body of the top vertebrae moves backwards, compared to the vertebral body below. Usually it happens because of degenerative changes of the vertebral disc or facet joints, however it can also be due to trauma. The loss of vertebral height and facet arthrosis cause a backward shifting. This movement can narrow the neural foraminal canal and compress the exiting nerve root, especially if the posterior longitudinal ligament or disc compresses the nerve root.

Retrolisthesis is graded either by a measurement in millimeters or grade level: I, II, III, or IV, with IV being the most severe. A study found that retrolisthesis at L5-S1 was 23.2%. Retrolisthesis combined with posterior degenerative changes was 4.8%, degenerative disc disease 16%, and vertebral endplate changes 4.8%. Age, sex, race, smoking, or education level did not affect the likelihood of developing retrolisthesis, compared to those with normal sagittal alignment.

Advancing age does increase the likelihood of developing vertebral endplate degenerative changes and disc disease, but it does not mean that a person will develop retrolisthesis. https://www.ncbi.nlm.nih.gov/pmc/articles/PMC2278018/

What Is Anterolisthesis?

Anterolisthesis is the forward movement of a vertebrae compared to the one below it. It can often occur as a child with excessive activity that damages the vertebrae and allows it to shift forward. Eventually, this area becomes solid and does not deteriorate later in life. The condition also develops with trauma in adulthood.

Movement is also graded on a scale of I, II, III, and IV. Mild-to-moderate anterolisthesis is usually treated with conservative therapy. Severe cases may require surgery for stabilization.

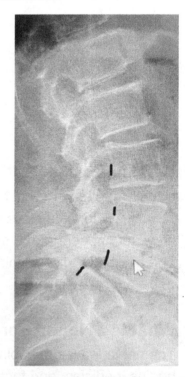

Are All Bulges Bad?
No. Damage to lumbar discs can produce small disc bulges. Small disc bulges found on many MRIs do not cause pain. However, a small bulge can create significant pain. This is why MRIs can reveal the structure, but do not accurately describe the function or pain levels.

Does A Disc Bulge Pinch The Nerve?
Kind of. Compression either results from direct compression by the disc extrusion or inflammation from the injury. The nerve is the softest thing that travels through the neural foraminal canal, and any additional material in the canal compresses the nerve. Nerve compression leads to pain, numbness, and tingling down the leg.

Hip Bursitis & Tendinopathy
Improper back mechanics causes excessive strain on the hip muscles and tendon attachments at the femur. This strain leads to tendon injuries (tendinopathy) or bursitis; irritated fluid filled sacs that allow tendons to glide across bone with less friction. These are common chronic injuries in patients with back pain. Video Hip Bursitis & Treatment

Arthritis Is the Second Biggest Concern and Excuse
Blaming all your back pain on arthritis is similar to blaming the neighbor kids for all neighborhood problems. Arthritic changes can cause pain, but are typically not the sole cause. It is easy for providers to point to arthritis on an X-ray and say "That is the source of your pain." Damage to bones does not occur independently; other tissues in the body have been absorbing the same forces and suffering damage, as well.

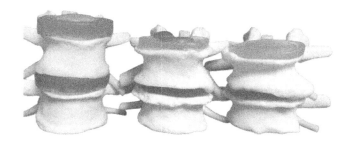

Is It Always Arthritis?

Back pain can result from pain sensors in the discs, joints, muscles, tendons, and ligaments in the lower back. Arthritic changes to the spine increase the likelihood of flare ups and make it easier to aggravate the joints with sitting and standing. Arthritis gets blamed as the source of pain, but it is not the only source of pain in the lower back. People with a history of low back pain typically have weakness in their core muscles and have created damage to their back ligaments and tendons. Daily stress and strain aggravate these tissues and send pain signals to the brain.

Video: Causes of Joint Pain

Is There a Cure?

Arthritis cannot be cured, but it *can* be managed. The trick is balancing core strength, endurance, flexibility, and neuromuscular control to stabilize the low back. Spinal decompression treatment can reduce pain and improve healing. Rehabilitation maintains those gains and reduces the shearing forces that produce pain and further degenerate the low back.

What are Muscles, Tendons, & Ligaments?

Tendons attach muscles to bone and have a better blood supply than ligaments. Tendons are responsible for transferring the contractile forces from muscles to bone. When muscles contract, they shorten and pull the bone on the other side of a joint, producing movement.

Ligaments are denser than tendons and have a limited blood supply. This is why when we stretch, tear, or damage a ligament, it takes much longer to heal. The poor blood supply means fewer nutrients are going to the ligaments and thus, prolonging recovery.

Muscles come in a variety of shapes and sizes. Some are very explosive and others more for endurance. The location of a muscle and its attachment sites are important in giving the muscle a mechanical advantage and producing specific movements across a joint. The tendon's attachment relative to the joint creates levers to aid in movement. As a general rule, any muscle that crosses a joint affects its movement. Muscles can either be the prime mover or simply help stabilize the joint.

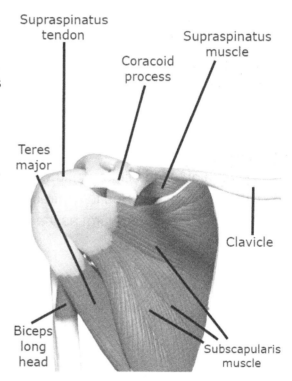

The term muscle fiber describes the individual units that make up muscle. There are two major types that slide past each other during contraction. The sliding of fibers creates an overall shortening of the muscle and the two tendon attachments are pulled closer together as the joint moves.

Muscle fibers contract with other fibers to create movement. The more muscle fibers the brain recruits to contract, the more force can be produced. The more fiber is used, the stronger it becomes by thickening and adding more fibers to each muscle cell.

A well-trained and used muscle gets bigger and stronger, and can handle more physical stress. Meanwhile, an inactive muscle begins to atrophy, or get smaller as the fibers are broken down and removed from the muscle cell.

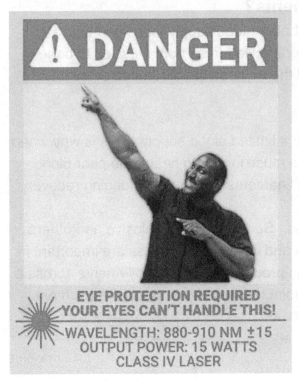

An example of a well-trained individual is on the safety sign in front of the laser room door.

That was obviously a picture of young Mike. Ten years ago I saw Mike shake a full five-gallon paint bucket above his shoulder like he was shaking a martini. At the end of the book are pictures of him doing some advanced shoulder exercises because he was the only one in the office who could do them.

How Muscle Contraction Works

Look at your right hand and straighten your fingers. Place your left hand onto muscles on the inside of the right elbow. Curl your fingers and flex the wrist toward the bicep muscles. The contraction of the finger and wrist flexor muscles are shortening and pulling the fingers and wrist in flexion. The muscle contraction can be felt by the fingers on your left hand.

To straighten the fingers and wrist, the body tells the wrist flexor muscles to relax and the extensor muscles to contract. The extensor muscle contraction can be felt on the other side of the forearm as the wrist and fingers extend.

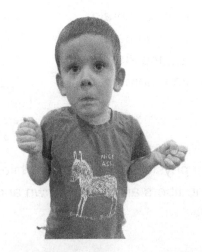

Max flexing like Uncle Mike

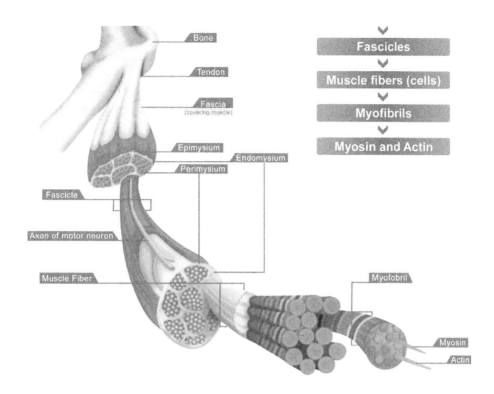

Concentric & Eccentric Muscle Contraction

Concentric contraction is when muscle fibers shorten to cause joint movement and lessen the joint angle. Eccentric contractions is when muscle fibers are lengthening under tension and allowing the joint angle to increase. The biceps muscles work together to produce flexion and extension of the elbow, often by using *concentric* and *eccentric* muscle contraction at the elbow joint.

For example, the bicep goes through concentric contraction when you flex your arm doing a biceps curl. Shortening muscle fibers are decreasing the elbow angle. Eccentric contraction occurs in the bicep muscle when slowly lowering the arm from the top of the curl back to the starting position. The bicep muscle is allowing the fibers to lengthen with the weight and increasing the elbow angle.

While most people focus on concentric motion when they strength train, it is actually the eccentric motion that is more likely to cause injuries. Eccentric contractions are harder on the muscle and the forces are greater. Ever go on a hike and wake up really sore two days later? Hiking uphill was mostly concentric muscle contraction, meanwhile the downhill was mostly eccentric on the quadriceps and calf muscles. Forty-eight hours after the hike, the delayed onset muscle soreness sets in from the eccentric muscle damage.

In therapy, we can use eccentric contraction to enhance recovery and build more supportive fibers than if we just used concentric contraction. More on that later.

Joints Are NOT the Only Source of Pain

Damage to joints does not happen without damaging the surrounding soft tissues. Chronic joint damage produces excessive strain to the tendons and ligaments that surround and protect the joint. The body attempts to protect the joints by overwhelming the protective soft tissues, which can heal and repair better than joints.

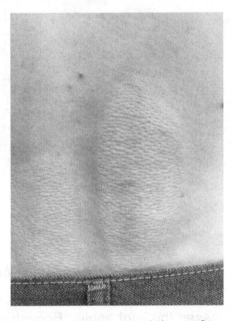

A great example of this involves the thumb. I cannot count the number of people who have told me they have arthritis in their thumb and nothing can be done about it. After a few weeks of treating their hands and thumb muscles with Graston, Shockwave, Class IV laser, and electric, their thumb feels better than it has in years. The treatments did not improve the bone damage; instead, it improved the soft tissue injuries around the thumb. Much of the pain they were feeling was from the soft tissue, not the arthritic joint.

Degeneration of the joints creates one type of pain, while chronic damage to ligaments and tendons creates another type of pain. The location of pain and aggravating factors are different for joints and soft tissues.

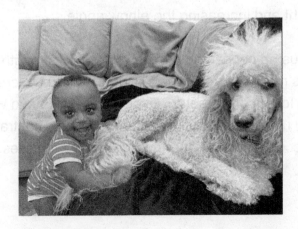

I'm Old, That Is the Way It Works

I have seen 80-year-olds with incredible core strength and minimal pain. On the other hand, I have seen 30-year-olds in terrible shape. There are some 1950s cars in great shape, and there are some 2015 models that are worn out.

One of my favorite patients has been extremely active throughout his life with running, tennis, and swimming. He was in his early 80s with an episode of acute low back pain. He was in a considerable amount of pain and a little reluctant to tell the story.

That morning he was swimming his usual one mile in the pool; three additional times per week he swims two miles. A younger woman was in the lane next to him and struck up a conversation just as he was finishing. She was very impressed that he could swim that much every week, and that he looked so good for his age.

He had a huge grin on his face the entire time he was telling the story. After a few more minutes of talking, she continued swimming down the lane. Charles said, "So at this point I'm feeling good about myself from the swim, and the young 50-year-old tells me I look good. My chest is all puffed up and I feel 20 years younger. That's when I decided to jump out of the pool instead of using the ladder on the edge. Going to the ladder is for old guys."

He was not going to push himself out of the pool backwards; he was going to jump out of the pool like a kid. He started with two hands pushing upward on the ledge as his right foot came out of the water to land on the ledge by his hands. As his body weight shifted to his leg, he knew he was in trouble. With all his might, he leaned forward to get both legs underneath him and shuffle to the men's locker room.

"The only thing I could think of was, 'Don't fall backward in the pool or let her see me lying in pain on the pool deck after her compliments.' So I made it to the locker room and laid on a bench for 30 minutes before coming straight to your office."

With a super big grin he said, "It doesn't matter how old you are; guys will always do stupid things to impress pretty ladies."

Video:

How to Avoid Low Back Pain

Spinal Curvatures

The body is trying to balance body weight and maintain a center of gravity. It uses spinal curves to absorb much of these forces. Think of a spring or slinky. The spring absorbs the forces and springs back up. If the spring is stretched or bent the wrong direction, the force absorption changes and certain areas will absorb too much force leading to damage.

The body has opposite curves to balance the forces. The cervical and lumbar spine curves are known as lordotic curves, while the thoracic and sacrum have kyphotic curves.

If the cervical spine begins to straighten and the head is pushed forward, the cervical lordotic curve decreases and increased stress is placed on the lower cervical spine. This postural change leads to increased lower cervical spine degeneration. The spring can't perform as designed. Forward head carriage leads to increased cervical and thoracic spinal degeneration, and also changes the position of the scapula leading to increased risk of shoulder injuries.

Think of a sloucher, rounded upper back and shoulders causing the head to move forward. The further the head moves the forward the greater the thoracic kyphotic curve becomes. The body is a system and changes in one area effects multiple regions and joints.

Increased thoracic kyphosis changes how the thoracic spine can extend and rotate, which affects shoulder movements. A person with a very pronounced kyphotic thoracic curve has to "hike their shoulders extra" to reach the cabinet shelf. The loss of rotation changes basic movement patterns and especially recreational sports. A golfer loses their ability to rotate the thoracic spine, leading to changes in their swing mechanics to compensate.

Changes to the thoracic and cervical spine create changes in how the upper back and neck muscles work to keep the head upright. The upper trapezius and levator scapula muscle work harder and harder to keep the head up. This leads to scapular elevation and rotation, which changes the glenohumeral position. This is the upper cross syndrome and SICK scapula discussed in greater detail within this book.

Kyphosis and Hyperkyphosis

Kyphosis is an increased forward curvature. In the thoracic spine an extreme kyphosis is often referred to as a hunchback, or round back. Older individuals with degenerative changes, osteoporotic fractures, or spinal stress fractures can develop the "Dowager hump," or patients refer to it as "back like my grandma," which is an extreme kyphosis because of spinal changes.

An increased thoracic kyphosis is associated with upper cross syndrome, the upper trapezius elevating and rotating the scapula. The pectoralis minor is pulling the scapula forward and rounding the shoulders. This position alters the glenohumeral joint position in a negative way. It increases the strain on soft tissues and likelihood of tissue rubbing or compressing with movements.

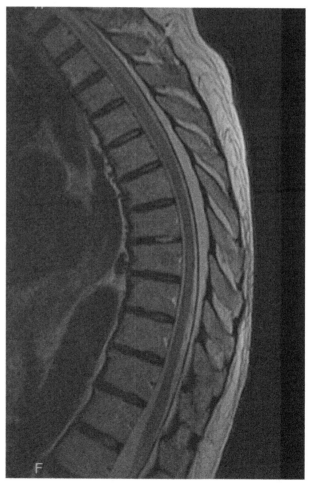

Secondly, this scapular starting position makes it difficult to reach above the head. The lower trapezius and rhomboid are unable to rotate the scapula upward. The compromised glenohumeral position is unable to rotate the humerus above the head and people compensate by hiking their shoulders to gain arm elevation. This poor movement pattern places increased stress on the shoulder soft tissues and frequently causes impingement syndromes.

The lack of thoracic extension is frequently compensated by shoulder hiking and increased lumbar extension for shoulder movements. Instead of extending the thoracic spine, people extended the torso through the lumbar and pelvic joints tipping the torso up.

Kyphosis is more common in women than men, particularly post-menopausal women who may have osteopenia (reduced bone density) or osteoporosis (even more bone loss). Both increase the risk of spinal stress fractures.

A loss of bone density in the thoracic vertebral bodies increases the risk of compression or insufficiency fractures. As the front of the body is "crushed" the overall height decreases leading to further kyphosis. Multiple compression fractures makes this situation even worse.

Once again, the body is a system and changes to the spine will affect the shoulder. Furthermore, weakness in the spine and core can lead to debilitating conditions over time. Work on your posture and core strength to avoid injuries.

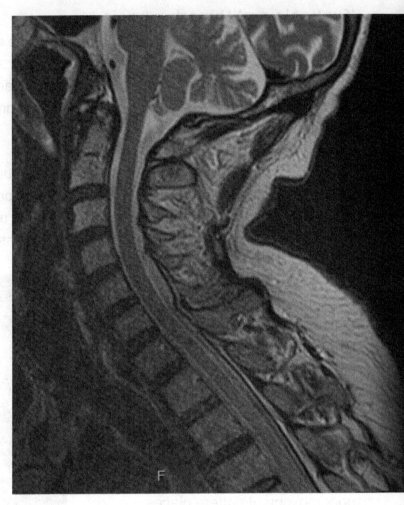

Scoliosis

Scoliosis is a lateral curvature of the spine that some individuals develop during childhood and adolescence. The degree of the curvature determines its treatment. A few degrees of thoracic tilt is expected to compensate for the heart. When the curvature is less than 10 degrees it is considered within normal limits. Between 10-20 degrees providers watch children to monitor changes. Getting above 20 degrees is problematic and above 40 degrees surgical intervention is considered. Getting to 40 degrees and above is severe and is more aggressively treated with bracing and surgery.

After skeletal maturity, there are not a lot of treatments that can be done to improve scoliosis besides not letting it get worse. The greater the scoliotic curves, the more emphasis a person should place on core strength, spinal stability, and posture. Increasing the wear and tear on the scoliotic curve accelerates the spinal degeneration.

Scoliosis causes spinal joints to rotate and laterally tip throughout the spinal column. This altered position changes how forces are distributed to the spinal column, often leading to facet or spinal disc degeneration at higher rates than a normal curvature.

Most people with mild scoliosis go throughout life without even noticing a difference. Moderate and severe scoliotic curves are much more problematic. The greater the scoliotic curve the more spinal rotation occurs and lateral flexion occurs. Essentially this alters the ability of the joints to rotate, flex, or extend, which leads to the body compensating above and below. As previously mentioned, compensating above or below leads to injuries and degeneration.

Individuals notice a "rib hump" where the rotated joints are most pronounced, especially compared to the other side. Moderate and severe scoliosis is commonly accompanied by upper cross and lower cross syndrome, which are not helping the long term situation.

For the shoulder, this means the thoracic spine cannot rotate or extend as well to help with normal scapula and humerus motion. Most individuals with moderate to severe scoliosis develop an increased kyphosis or forward-rounding shoulders. As mentioned in the previous section, an increased thoracic kyphosis alters glenohumeral joint positions and movements, leading to increased shoulder injuries.

For adults and older adults, scoliosis is trying to manage and limit additional degeneration. Exercises can focus on increasing spinal and scapular stabilization to limit degenerative changes. The level of scoliosis and spinal changes determines the starting point of exercises and stretches, and each individual has a different treatment plan for their functional ability.

When a person has shoulder injuries and scoliosis, the shoulder pain needs to be treated to decrease pain. Long term treatment and goals need to address the curvatures, spinal stability, and maintaining pain free joint range of motion throughout the spine.

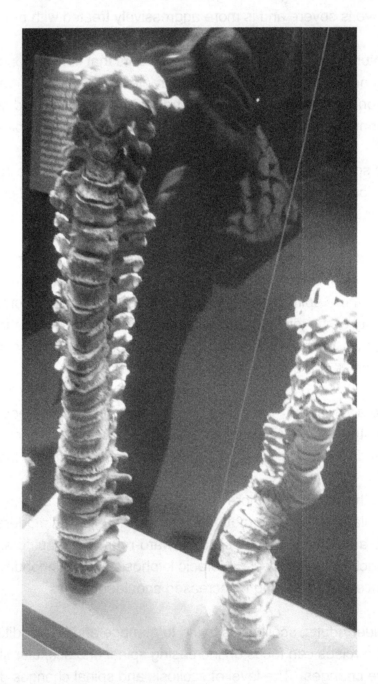

Chapter 3: Imaging

X-rays are an inexpensive and easy tool to enhance your treatment and expectations. X-ray images show the bones and the spaces between, arthritic changes, and stenosis. Changes to spinal curves are often seen, along with any metal from previous surgeries. Flexion and extension X-rays determine normal versus unstable spinal movements.

Unfortunately, X-rays do not show soft tissue changes, disc bulges, or disc herniations. They are not necessary for every patient or injury, but are often the initial diagnostic imaging tool utilized to rule out fractures.

After the initial examination, your provider will decide if you need X-rays to determine treatment. With certain criteria, a trial treatment plan can begin without imaging.

If the provider suspects, or needs to determine, how many discs are involved, he/she will utilize an MRI to evaluate if a disc is becoming dehydrated, bulging, or herniating. The radiologist can measure the size of a disc extrusion, which helps in determining the proper treatment plan.

Video: When to Get an MRI for Low Back Pain

When Is It Necessary to Get an MRI?

An MRI is a very useful tool for evaluating the vertebrae, discs, arthritis, and compression of the spinal cord or nerve roots. It will show an incredible amount of detail on the structure of the spine. MRIs can be helpful when used properly.

First of all, you should *not* get an MRI every time your back hurts. There are national guidelines for when to order an MRI for low back pain:
- Sudden onset of severe sciatica pain with loss of motor, sensory, or reflex.
- If the provider suspects something big and nasty is going, and wants to rule it out. Such as cancers or some fractures.
- Trauma that has produced radiating pain and loss of motor, sensory, or sensation.
- Loss of bowel or bladder function, and changing sensation in the groin area. Go to the Emergency Room and they will do an MRI to see if immediate surgical intervention is necessary.

For most low back episodes, the recommendation is six weeks of conservative therapy, then order an MRI if the person is not improving and/or symptoms worsen.

Orthopedic Tests and Nerve Root Compression

An MRI is not the only way to diagnose disc injuries and nerve root compressions. Several orthopedic tests performed by your provider can indicate whether something is compressing on the nerve or spinal cord. When a series of the tests are positive in a predictable pattern, then more-likely-than-not, you have a disc injury at a specific level.

For example, when Straight Leg Raise, Milgram's, Slump, and Valsalva tests all reproduce radiating pain down to the big toe, this indicates a disc injury. Weakness or loss of sensation on the big toe also indicates L5 nerve root compression. The combination of positive tests and symptom intensity gives your provider the information necessary for diagnosis.

Video

Sciatica - Differences Between Lumbar Disc
and Piriformis Syndrome - Diagnoses Error

Does a Really Bad MRI Require Surgery?

No. I have seen some really bad MRIs that produce minimal low back pain. I have seen small disc extrusions produce severe pain, motor loss, and require surgery.

If a person is responding to conservative treatment, the best course of action is to keep going with treatment. If a person is getting worse with conservative treatment, I suggest advanced treatments such as pain management injections. If a person continues to get worse after the injections, it might be time to consider surgery.

Severe lower back pain with sciatica does not mean surgery is necessary; most symptoms will improve with conservative treatments. A few will not improve and will benefit from surgery.

In the area around the spinal cord (central spinal canal), there is some extra room. If the disc extrusion is not compressing too much on the spinal cord or nerve root, the patient has options for conservative therapy management. When the disc extrusion is causing significant compression, a trial of conservative treatment is recommended; however, with deteriorating symptoms surgery might be the best course of action.

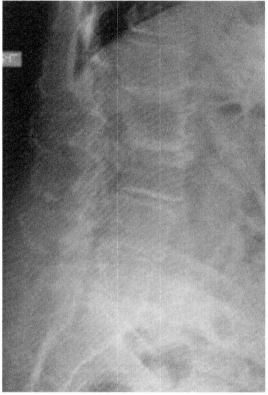

Last year I had a 35-year-old male who had a really large disc extrusion on the L5 nerve root. He was in a lot of pain and could not sit, stand, walk, or drive for longer than a few minutes. He really did not want to get surgery for personal reasons.

He suffered for nine months. His home and work life were significantly compromised. It took months for his disc extrusion to shrink in size and shift away from the nerve root. He very slowly was able to regain core strength, endurance, and daily back function. He was exceptionally diligent in his daily activities, exercises, and eventually core strengthening. He fought through every day for the first few months before seeing improvement.

His story is an example that a person can choose his treatment path but has to be willing to endure the consequences.

Video:

How to Avoid Back Surgery

Chapter 4: Just Getting it Done

The low back is part of a complex system for movement. Posture and positioning of joints is as important as the muscular movement patterns themselves. Just because you can swing a golf club or reach above your head doesn't mean you do it well or without tissue compromise.

I call this the driver's license principle. Just because you have a driver's license doesn't mean you are a good driver. Bad drivers can still drive on the roads. How many people do you know who think they are a good driver but really aren't?

Just because you can move doesn't mean you move it well.

Patients struggle with overcoming poor posture and movement patterns. Many people view movement as something automatic. They *never consider how well they move until something hurts.*

When a patient thinks about getting the box of cereal out of the cabinet, their only concern is whether their hand is able to reach the box on the top shelf. From a provider standpoint, we want to look at how well the thoracic spine extends. Is the scapula in the correct initial positions? Does elevation of the arm, clavicle, and scapula occur at appropriate times? Does the patient hike the shoulder up in order to elevate the arm? Is the upper trapezius overactive, leading to excessive elevation and rotation of the scapula? Is the position and movements of the glenohumeral joint appropriate? Is the low back supported or is the person extending too much?

Improper movements and muscle coordination leads to excessive strain and eventual soft tissue injuries and pain.

Once again, a patient only cares about being able to reach the box of their heart-healthy cereal. A provider cares about how well the shoulder, back, and pelvis functions in order to reach the cereal, and if these movements are leading to improper positions and future injuries.

This reinforces the importance of the provider and a patient having a clear agreement on a treatment plan to reach the patient's goals. I realize that most people are past the stage of life where throwing a fastball is a priority. However, everyone needs to be able to reach the top shelf of the kitchen pantry and pick up a shoe without pain.

I hope this book will provide valuable information to help get you out of pain today while also preventing future injuries.

It is not just about getting the movement done. It is about doing it well.

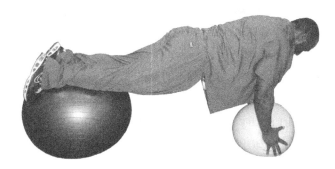

Managing Stress and Strain

After the pain levels decrease, the trick is to avoid excessive stress and strain by increasing your activity levels *slowly*. Every joint in the body is capable of handling a certain amount of stress on a daily and weekly basis.

Applying more stress than the weakest tissue can handle will lead to injury.

Not all tissue can handle the same stress loads, nor is every muscle equally strong. Rehabilitation is working through a process of getting all the tissues ready to handle stress forces, and all of the muscles strong enough to perform the activity.

It is unrealistic to expect that you can return to your pre-injury level of activity right away. The motto here is, "Start low and go slow. Prove you can and then do a little more."

Tissue adapts to handle specific types of stress and strain placed upon them. When an individual applies an unfamiliar stress or in an awkward position, injuries are more likely to occur.

Proximal Stability Leads to Distal Mobility

The body requires a solid base to perform optimally. If the foundation - in this case the body's stabilizer musculature - is weak, a person cannot produce or transfer forces efficiently. I like to use the example of trying to shoot a cannon from a canoe. Without a solid base the cannonball will not travel as far or be as accurate.

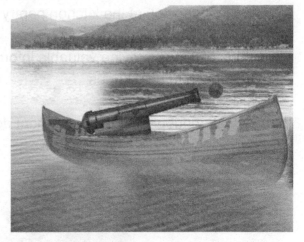

Upper cross syndrome changes the scapular position, which then alters shoulder, elbow, wrist, and hand movements. Swinging a club or racquet once or twice probably won't be a problem, but trying to swing the racquet 50 times from a dysfunctional base leads to excessive stress and strain in the elbow. This is an example of creating an injury with repetitive movements from a poor mechanical position. More on this topic later.

In some cases, treatment can focus only on the injured muscles and tendons. If we get the pain and inflammation to decrease and encourage proper tissue remodeling, then the problem goes away. In this case, we only had to remove a few handful of pennies from the jar to solve the problem. It is great when this works and the case is easy.

Unfortunately, sometimes the injury will not go away or quickly returns when resuming activity. In these cases, treatment cannot focus on only what hurts, especially for chronic conditions. We often need to look above and below the pain and address the causes of excessive soft tissue strain. Therapies also need to address breaking down the improper tissue healing and restoring proper healing, as described below in the treatment section.

Paying the Piper

We ask our low back to do a lot through the years. It should not be unexpected that at some point we throw too many pennies in the jar, and this very remarkable structure becomes overwhelmed. Realistically, it is amazing the back functioned pain-free as long as it did. Most of us have challenged our muscles, but did very little to enhance their strength and function with stretching, massage therapy, or protective rehabilitation exercises.

This book will discuss the most common injuries and treatments, but it is only a guide. Obviously we recommend you get properly diagnosed by a provider with a great understanding of the musculoskeletal system, and not using a combination of Crazy Uncle Joe and Dr. Google.

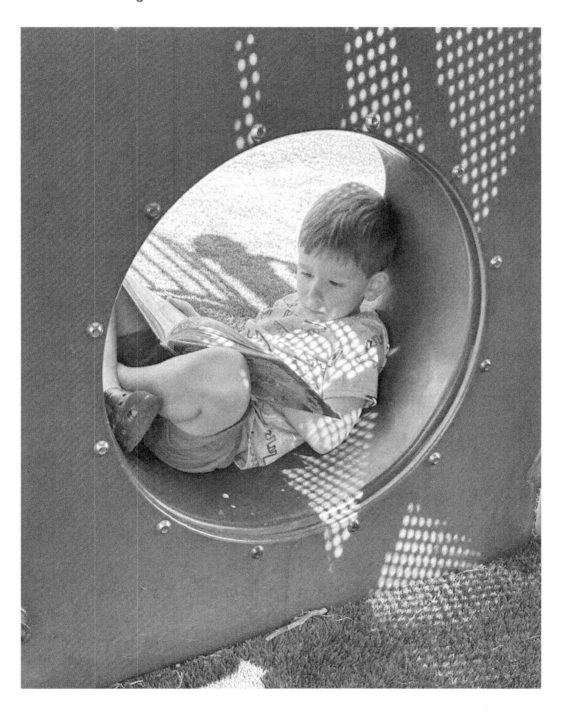

Find a comfortable spot and keep reading the best low back book you have ever read (and only one)!

Chapter 5: Chronic Low Back Pain

Here is your sign!!!!!
Comedian Bill Engvall had a skit about dumb decisions people make that would end with "Here's your sign." I have earned that joke more than a few times.

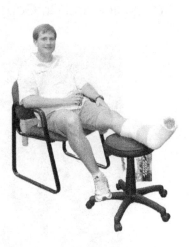

Chronic low back pain also shows a few signs:
- Increasing stiffness
- Increasing dull and sharp pain
- Waking up stiffer
- More soreness when standing for prolonged periods of time
- Increased pain riding in the car
- Repeated bending leads to pain
- Certain chairs aggravate your back
- Increased pain with walking, bending, twisting, or reaching

The above are all signs that your low back health is deteriorating. Making good decisions about exercises, stretches, treatments, and avoiding aggravating activities will help you move in the right direction and keep you from having to lie on your back on the tile floor.

Video:
Why Most People Have Chronic Back Pain

The Biggest Reason People Have Chronic Low Back Pain
They focus exclusively on pain. When patients have chronic low back pain, they often judge their back health on pain. If it doesn't hurt then their back is great, similar to judging how well a car performs based on how it looks sitting in the driveway. If it's clean and the tires are full of air then it must be well maintained and drive smoothly. A ridiculous statement, but it is similar to judging lower back health according to pain levels.

Pain is the last symptom to develop and the first to go away, which is why pain cannot be used to evaluate lower back health.

The Second Biggest Reason People Have Chronic Low Back Pain

They stop working on function and spinal stability when the back pain disappears. As a result, they lose strength, leading to pain in the future. This is obvious but happens every day.

Video:
Muscle Fatigue Leads to Injuries

The Third Biggest Reason People Have Chronic Low Back Pain

People fail to continue challenging themselves with harder exercises. Those individuals who continue with their home exercises often perform the same ones as when they stopped treatment. They fail to further develop and challenge their spinal stabilization; in other words, they are doing enough to prevent a backslide, but nothing more.

Returning to climbing the mountain comparison, performing the same exercises will only keep a person at the same level. They won't climb higher towards achieving a better quality of life; they are just doing enough not to slide backwards.

Chronic lower back pain is the result of years of dysfunction. A person's functional level slowly slides downhill for a variety of reasons. Most people become motivated to change their habits and commit to improvement when they hit rock bottom. Unfortunately, the bottom is a long way from the top. Does it seem realistic that a month's worth of exercises will restore all of the functional weakness and compensations?

In summary, people fail to improve because:
1. **Focus on avoiding pain**
2. **Stop doing the exercises that helped them to improve**
3. **Fail to continue challenging their systems to reach maximal improvement**

Before I produced these books and educational email, I had the two following examples hanging on the physical therapy wall. It reminded us to communicate, set proper goals, and understand the progression.

Pain Progression Example
This is an example of a patient's pain progression descending from worst to best.

- *Constant* sharp pain with *frequent* severe stabbing pain.
- *Constant* dull pain with *occasional* sharp stabbing pain.
- *Occasional* stiffness, mostly dull ache with *infrequent* sharp stabbing pain with movement.
- *Frequent* stiffness, *occasional* dull ache, and *infrequent* mildly sharp pain with movement.
- *Occasional* stiffness and *occasional* dull pain.
- Mostly good but with *infrequent* stiffness and *infrequent* dull ache after increased activity.
- *Infrequent* tightness and stiffness, but mostly without any discomfort.
- No pain.

Healing is a progression of rebuilding broken tissue, similar to adding fiber to a rope to make it bigger and stronger. Strengthening occurs in the muscles around the injured area. This is not a quick process, and I assure you this takes longer than you would like. It is similar to going to the gym and exercising; seven runs on the treadmill will not make you fast.

Notice the above pain progression does not correlate to any specific function or activity. Pain can improve and the function may still be awful. Sometimes the two improve together. Usually pain improves first and functional improvement follows.
This is why **_I care more about function than pain_**. How well the joint complex and surrounding area functions determines your long term *risk of injury*.

Goals Of Treatment Example

Goals of treatment............**Your** goals are **our** goals! You chose what they are.
1. Get you out of pain.
2. Improve your function (50% of possible improvement).
3. Reduce your risk of reinjury (70% of possible).
4. Maximize functional improvement (90%).
5. As good as we can reasonably get.

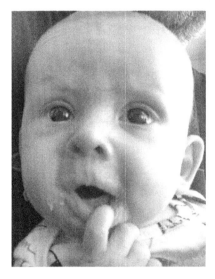

You choose the level of improvement you want to reach. We understand that not everyone has the time or desire to reach Goal #5, and that's okay. If you tell us your goal is #2, we will develop a plan that gets you to #2 as quickly as possible. It is okay to change your goals mid treatment; just tell us.

One of my favorite patient stories is described in the video below. He thought people with low back pain were babies and faking it. Then he started having back problems which changed his perspective and approach.

People who experience chronic back pain have a different outlook on life, function, pain, expectations, and fear of future injuries.

Video: I Thought People With Low Back Pain Were Babies

Why Doesn't Everyone Have Back Pain

In a retirement community, everyone has a lot of miles on their low back, but why doesn't everyone have low back pain? What makes them different? There are many different factors, but one of the **biggest factors is the ability to absorb and create forces**.

Sitting, standing, walking, bending, twisting, swinging a club, or changing directions on a tennis court all involve producing forces and absorbing those forces without producing injuries.

Baseball is About Producing Forces and Absorbing Forces

I heard a trainer for the Atlanta Braves talk about baseball injuries. He said, "baseball is about producing force and absorbing force." I believe the same concept occurs in the low back. Every movement produces forces on the low back, which also requires the back to absorb forces.

When the core cannot properly absorb daily forces excessive strain damages the spine, tendons, ligaments, and muscles. A weak core leads to increased damage. A strong core absorbs the forces and protects the back.

Learn to produce and absorb force in the low back again!

Video:

Pelvis Stability and Pitcher Injury Study

CrossFit With Your Grandson

This year I had a patient with a knee injury from performing box jumps at CrossFit. Knee pain happens frequently with jumping and squatting activities. The unusual part of the story is that my patient went to CrossFit with his grandson. My patient obviously is in great shape. A lifetime of exercise allowed him to perform explosive activity in his "close to retirement age."

He was obviously the oldest person in the class, and enjoyed spending time with his grandson in a unique environment.

His core and back muscles are incredibly strong and he is well coordinated. He produces and absorbs forces very well. His lifetime of hard work has paid off, and he continues to exercise daily at a high level.

I am not encouraging everyone to go to CrossFit or perform plyometrics with their grandchildren. I think it is incredible what the body can do with proper training, at any age.

Senior Olympics Sprinter

My last year of chiropractic school I was interning at a clinic in the Florida panhandle. I would like to say I went to Florida for the educational experience, but after three Minneapolis winters I absolutely went for the white sandy beaches. My clinic was a mile from the beach, and you could smell the ocean from the parking lot. It was so much better than the Minneapolis winter.

The clinic had me treat all athletic patients. Beth, the office manager, handed me a file of a runner with a shoulder injury. She said he made it very clear that "he was not a runner or jogger but a sprinter!" Beth gave me a very clear warning, do not say "jogging or running;" he was a 75-year-old sprinter.

When I opened the treatment room door, I immediately apologized to the 50ish-age man for being in the wrong room. After Beth confirmed it was the correct room, I went back in to talk to Mr. Johnson. He was actually 75 but looked to be in his 50's. He hurt his shoulder sprinting up and down hills, training for the Senior Olympics.

It was really fun talking to Mr. Johnson. He was a decent sprinter in high school and joined a track group again in his 50s after needing an athletic outlet. Mr. Johnson had significant success through the years, and this was an important year.

He often would place between fifth and eighth in the Senior Olympic sprints. He was moving into the older age division, so he was going to be the "young sprinter" this year! This was his year to place in the top three and he didn't want his shoulder injury affecting his training.

Years of athletic endeavors kept him in great shape. It was a great experience meeting a 75-year-old sprinter and helping him with his training.

Video: Half Marathon Runner with Lower Leg Pain

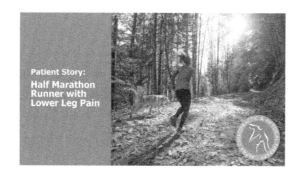

Sitting & Back Pain

Why Is Sitting So Bad for Discs and Low Back Pain?
Discs require movement for blood flow and nutrients. Sitting in a static position comprises the disc and slows blood flow. Think of a wet sponge; discs receive blood by taking a foot of the sponge and having fluid rush inward. Stepping on the sponge pushes fluid out. Sitting is like half compressing an edge of the sponge for hours.

Video: Conrad & Fogerty Exercise Theories

All I Did Was Sit
Every year my dad drives from Montana down to sunny Arizona for the winter. He is always surprised that his lower back hurts after driving 22 hours in the car over two days. His statement is always the same: "all I did was sit." He didn't think it would be too hard or traumatic on his lower back to sit.

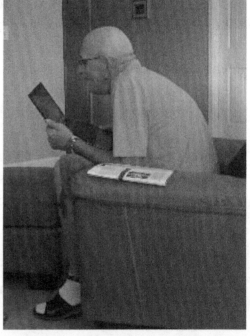

Every year he forgets that he is older, arthritic, and not as strong as he used to be. His lower back flares up for a week or two, and then he forgets until the next trip. He spends two weeks complaining about his back and learning the exact same exercises as the previous year, that he conveniently forgot.

The combination of long hours, poor posture, and lack of core strength produces a lower back injury every year. Combining two days of driving with unpacking the car, getting the house ready, and catching up on yard work guarantees an injury.

Poor posture and seating positions overwhelms the tissue, leading to injury. He could manage the trauma to his lower back if he took three days to drive down instead of two. He should take more breaks along the way. Ideally he would have better strength and flexibility before the trip, but that would take consistency and commitment.

Dad Earned His Low Back Pain Through Sitting

As with many people his age, my dad claims to have been athletic in his youth. Then family, desk jobs, and finally computer work took its toll. His exercise levels were minimal for many years, and his waist line required new belts every few years.

The modern lifestyle of prolonged sitting and lack of exercise contributes to lower back pain. The body loses essential strength and neuromuscular control and begins to compensate with the wrong muscles. Continued sitting further exacerbates this problem, leading to increased joint shearing and strain with movement.

This progression of back pain from prolonged sitting was explained very well in an article written by Christine Lynders PT, published in HSS Journal August 2019, titled "The Critical Role of Development of the Transverse Abdominis in the Prevention and Treatment of Low Back Pain."
https://www.ncbi.nlm.nih.gov/pmc/articles/PMC6778169/pdf/11420_2019_Article_9717.pdf

> It is known that prolonged sitting is detrimental to the maintenance of proper spinal alignment and stability, but mechanical loading of the spine during sitting and standing is still not well understood. A commonly cited 1970 study by Nachemson and Elfstrom found that with standing there is approximately 100-kg compression on the spinal discs and that with sitting these forces increase to approximately 140 kg and rise further to 185 kg with forward bending while seated [18]. Lifting an object from that forward seated position can increase those loads to 220 kg [16, 18].
>
> We have also come to understand that prolonged sitting causes lumbar flexion, reversing normal lordosis and leading to increased compressive, static (segmental) loading over time [3]. Callaghan and McGill also found that sitting results in significantly higher compressive loads in the low back than standing does [3]. Spinal structure is designed to maintain upright posture, absorb shock, and accommodate bipedal gait through three normal curves: cervical lordosis, thoracic kyphosis, and lumbar lordosis.
>
> Spinal alignment also depends on stabilizing structures such as the facet joints, spinal ligaments, and the intervertebral discs, as well as the muscles that provide dynamic stability by absorbing the energy of loading the spine during activities.

The author further describes the critical role of activating the transverse abdominis muscle and the deep spinal stabilizers to protect, stabilize, and retrain proper movements, thus avoiding lower back pain. In her clinic, she likes to use the phrase "suck it in" to describe activating the transverse abdominis muscle. She encourages patients to "suck it in" throughout the day whenever they bend forward to brush their teeth or pick something off the ground. She wants people to find ways to consciously trigger the transverse abdominis with normal activities until it becomes a subconscious action.

So start sucking it in throughout the day. You can tell people it isn't to look good, it's for your back health.

Why Does It Hurt Getting Out of a Chair?
Leaning forward to stand shifts the weight load to the front of discs, pushing forces backward against the injured disc. Stress loads are shifting through the spine and loading different parts of the back during the sit-to-stand transition. You will feel pain when the stress shifts to the injured tissue.

EVOLUTION OF THE DESK JOB
THAT GIVES YOU BACK ACHE AND DEPRESSION

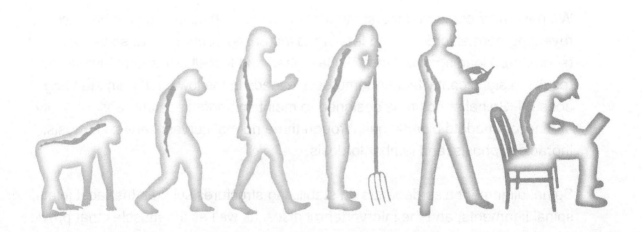

I Am Almost Always Wrong

As providers, we are more often wrong than correct with our initial shoulder diagnosis and treatment plans. Yes, I did just say that. Initial plan A is almost always wrong in the low back. Treatment plans always move to plan B, C, D, E, F, and G. Chronic low back pain never recovers in a linear fashion.

The back's complexity and all of the moving parts involved in its dysfunction make it necessary to constantly modify and change treatment strategies. The plan will shift as a person improves, or the next weak link in the kinetic chain is identified. This is why exercises cannot be provided on a worksheet to be performed at set intervals. A good provider understands that each patient is unique and will improve at their own rate.

Adding the appropriate exercises at the appropriate time is the most effective plan. I think it's safe to say that no provider is so good at diagnosis that they can determine your exact treatment progression on the first visit, including the rehabilitative exercises.

As providers we need to treat your unique injury with a unique treatment plan. Most people have many of the same building blocks that need to be put into the treatment plan, but the timing of exercises and soft-tissue treatments will vary person to person.

This Drives Type A People Nuts

Type A patients like to have a very detailed plan of exactly when certain treatments are going to be initiated and performed, and how they will improve during the course of these treatments. It can be a little frustrating for these people who want a set of answers up front, but unfortunately, that is simply not the way healing and injury treatment works.

A realistic low back treatment plan and improvement schedule tends to resemble the stock market with its day-to-day fluctuations. A steady trend of improvement can be followed by a few crazy up and down days, then suddenly jump back to previous levels. Sometimes these wild fluctuations are due to a known cause or concern, and other times they occur for no apparent reason. This is the way treatment goes.

Kids These Days

Kids these days. It amazes me how many kids (and their parents and even grandparents) get their news and information from social media platforms. Many of these individuals have undying faith in treatment plans and rehabilitative exercises they find in Twitter posts, YouTube videos, and on Tik-Tok.

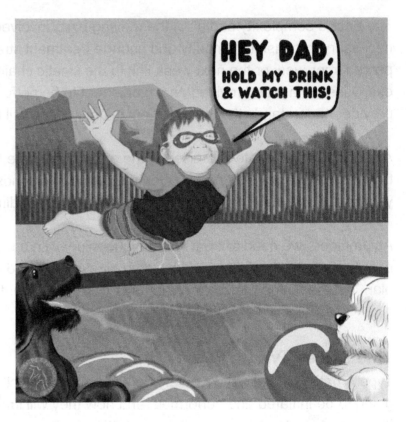

Surfing online platforms leads down a rabbit hole of quick fix videos and magical cures for pain, typically prefaced by phrases such as "solve your back pain with these four exercises" and "the most important back exercise." List stories are particularly popular, i.e. "the five most important," "ten most successful," etc. I have seen some pretty good clips and videos, but most of those are for young and basically healthy individuals. List stories don't work well for complex medical conditions, such as the typical chronic low back injury for an older adult.

I have not seen a video titled "Quickly and simply improve back pain for those with 60 years of wear and tear, anterior head carriage, forward shoulder rounding, scapular dyskinesis, lower cross syndrome, limited hip flexibility, and poor core stabilization." Such a video might actually be worth watching.

Google is a fantastic search engine, but it requires putting in the correct search criteria. That requires understanding the problem, in depth. It also requires being able to distinguish good quality information from bad, which isn't as easy as it looks.

It Wasn't Google's Fault

A 78-year-old patient came into the office with shoulder pain. He is in good shape and very active for his age, and had been golfing more and working around the house, which led to the shoulder pain. We have seen him for neck and back pain in the past. He has significantly elevated and forward-rounding shoulders, and is the classic picture of upper cross syndrome in the Sun Lakes retirement community. His thoracic spine (mid back) is very rounded and has significant degenerative changes.

He described his shoulder pain as very sharp when trying to lift his arm, localized to the front of the shoulder. He couldn't raise his hand above his head without intense stabbing pain. With a little help, he could lift his arm further and then the pain decreased. He didn't have any pain when his hand reached its highest point. Sleeping was very uncomfortable. Worst of all, it was affecting his golf game.

All of the orthopedic tests indicated a supraspinatus sprain and shoulder impingement. We treated him on a Saturday, trying to decrease the pain and muscle spasms. We showed him some light exercises and stretches to help, along with icing instructions. We quickly talked about shoulder pain progression and the treatment options for each stage. But the focus was on decreasing the sharp pain and inflammation, and reducing overuse. The patient needed to stop trying to fight through the pain.

With his posture and spinal degenerative changes, I would have expected to see more reports of neck, upper back, and shoulder pain. Fortunately for him, his musculoskeletal pain had been few and far between. *At least that's what he admitted to.*

On Monday he came into the office frustrated because the shoulder wasn't getting better. It was actually worse. He was 78 and never had a problem before, so why now? Secondly, why hadn't he gotten better? He had Googled a description of his symptoms and located a 10-page report on treatments along with exercises for frozen shoulder.

On Sunday he did all the frozen shoulder exercises. The instructions on the sheet said it was okay to have pain with the exercises, and that it was recommended to have discomfort during the movements.

Sigh......

As you can imagine, forcing the shoulder through the exercises flared up the injury.

This kind of thing happens all the time. My process was to perform the exam again, explaining again why his diagnosis was a shoulder impingement. I also reviewed orthopedic tests and movements that ruled out frozen shoulders. I then went through the shoulder exercises and pointed out which ones were similar to those I had given him on the previous visit. I also advised against performing certain exercises because they *would aggravate his shoulder.* The exercises in the Google article were intended to stretch and tear the capsule scar tissue, which would also compress his injured tissue: the worst thing he could do.

At the end he asked me if I was sure of my diagnosis or should he get a second opinion. I told him this was my most definite diagnosis all week. I was absolutely sure it wasn't a frozen shoulder.

He then asked, "why did my research find frozen shoulder and nothing about impingement?"

My response was: "Because you typed into the Google search box, 'can't raise my arm above my head'. You should have searched for 'pain lifting hand 90 to 120 degree angle - painful arc sign.' So it was 100% user error."

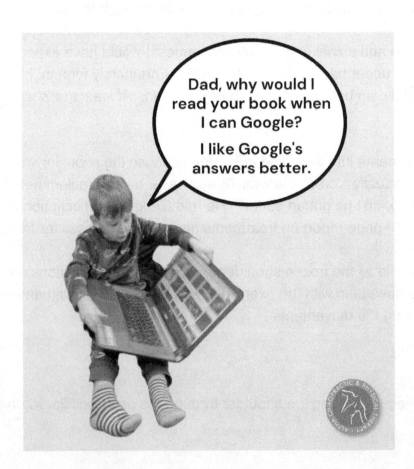

Walking and Back Pain

Why Is a Smooth Walking Gait Important?
An awkward Frankenstein's monster-type gait causes excessive pounding and strain on the knees, which is also sent upwards to the back. An awkward gait increases lower back flare ups and injuries. A smooth walking gait glides across the ground and forces are evenly distributed.

Changes in Walking Gait from Low Back Pain
Everyone has seen a person with severe low back pain walking through a grocery store; short, deliberate steps with a forward or sideways lean. The walking gait becomes very cautious and deliberate.

Not everyone returns to a normal walking gait when the pain disappears. An article published in April 2006 in the *European Spine Journal* evaluated how muscle activation and joint movement changes with chronic low back pain.

In, "Effects of Chronic Low Back Pain on Trunk Coordination and Back Muscle Activity During Walking: Changes in Motor Control," the authors concluded that people with chronic low back pain walk more slowly than people without pain. These people have increased erector spinae muscle activity (guarding). The lower back muscles remain tighter and restrict low back movement. Thoracic and pelvic rotational movements are also altered when walking.
https://www.ncbi.nlm.nih.gov/pmc/articles/PMC3454567/#__ffn_sectitle

People in the above study did not have active back pain. Their bodies continued to compensate from previous pain episodes by guarding and tightening the lower back muscles, resulting in altered joint movement patterns when walking.

This is exactly why we differentiate between pain and functional levels. Pain will disappear, but does the function return to proper levels? These patients benefit from stabilization and core training exercises, in order to restore proper movement patterns and reduce protective muscle guarding.

Altered Walking Gait from Low Back Pain

A 2006 study published in the *European Spine Journal* evaluated walking gait changes in patients with low back pain. The article "Effects of Chronic Low Back Pain on Trunk Coordination and Back Muscle Activity During Walking: Changes in Motor Control" investigated how people altered their walking gait with low back pain.
https://www.ncbi.nlm.nih.gov/pmc/articles/PMC3454567/

Walking gait was significantly compromised in patients with low back pain. The erector spinae (lower back muscles next to spine) became tighter and more active. Gait became more rigid and less fluid, along with changes to pelvic movements. People with low back pain also walked more slowly than those without pain.

Video:
Altered Gait Leads to Knee Pain

Balance and Chronic Back Pain

A person with chronic low back pain also loses balance and stability while standing and walking. For example, the ability to stabilize oneself when standing on one foot

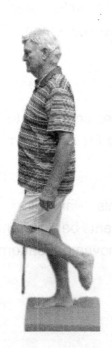

decreases with chronic low back pain. As a person's condition continues to deteriorate, the single leg stance stability worsens. The poor balance is a consequence of pain and poor proprioception from the low back facet joints, and weakness and loss of stability from the deep spinal stabilizer muscles.

This is not a new concept. A study published in 1998 in the journal *Spine* titled "One-Footed and Externally Disturbed Two-Footed Postural Control in Patients with Chronic Low Back Pain and Healthy Control Subjects: A Controlled Study with Follow Up" evaluated this principle.

The study concluded: "Postural stability is easily disturbed in case of impairment in strength, coordination, or effective coupling of muscles in the lumbar and pelvic area. Patients with chronic low back pain seem to experience impairment in these functions, which should be taken into consideration when back rehabilitation programs are planned." https://www.ncbi.nlm.nih.gov/pubmed/9794052

Building on the recommendations of the prior study, a 2018 study published in the *Journal of Exercise Rehabilitation*, "Comparison of the Effects of Stability Exercise and Balance Exercise on Muscle Activity in Female Patients with Chronic Low Back Pain," showed that back pain was reduced in both stability and balance exercise groups, through different mechanisms. https://www.ncbi.nlm.nih.gov/pmc/articles/PMC6323339/

A similar finding appeared in a 2018 study published in the *BMC Musculoskeletal Disorder Journal* titled "Postural Awareness and its Relationship to Pain: Validation of an Innovative Instrument Measuring Awareness of Body Posture in Patients with Chronic Pain." The study found that improving posture decreased spinal and shoulder pain. https://www.ncbi.nlm.nih.gov/pubmed/29625603

For this reason we combine traditional strengthening exercises with stability and balance exercises to reduce back pain and enhance spinal stability.

Video: Patient Case Study: Knee Pain with Arthritis and Treatment Options

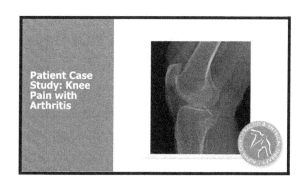

Watch the above video to learn about an older knee with pain and degeneration and see what we do to get it better.

It explains the anatomy, what we are looking for, and the treatment.

Additional Sources of Back Pain

Is Arthritis Pain Different Than Ligament Pain?
Absolutely. Degeneration of the joints creates one type of pain, while chronic damage to ligaments creates another type of pain. The location of pain and aggravating factors are different for joints and ligaments.

Video: Treating Tendon & Ligament Injuries

How Can Muscles, Tendons, and Ligaments Cause Pain?
When soft tissue does not heal correctly, scar tissue and adhesions develop. These create weak spots that flare up with mechanical stress. Every time a person overloads the weak spots, it creates pain. If the core muscles cannot stabilize the back, extra strain irritates the scar tissue patches.

Soft tissue treatments such as with shockwave therapy, class IV cold laser, and Graston Technique can help these weak spots heal.

Does Central Canal Stenosis Mean that I Will Have Chronic Pain Forever?
No. Mild central canal stenosis can create problems from time to time. Stenosis makes it more likely to have problems but does not always cause pain. Moderate central canal stenosis requires more effort to keep joints moving and reduce additional damage to the spine. People with moderate stenosis can maintain a high quality of life with proper movement activities and work.

Severe stenosis is trickier to manage. A person is more likely to have several bouts of pain a year. Most patients feel chronic stiffness and tightness on a daily basis. It is easier to trigger moderate and severe pain and takes longer to get rid of than in the past. Some patients respond very well to spinal injections or nerve ablation therapy.

What Is Central Canal Stenosis Versus Neural Foraminal Stenosis?
Stenosis of the central canal produces pain radiating down both legs because it compresses the spinal cord. Neuroforaminal stenosis compresses one nerve root and produces symptoms down one leg.

What Is Spinal Cord Compression?
This is typically caused by degenerative changes to the vertebral bodies, extending bone spurs backwards, or disc extrusions pushing onto the spinal cord. Chronic damage to the ligament that runs down the back of the vertebrae can also lead to stenosis. Disc bulges pushing backwards can also produce spinal cord compression.

Do Astronauts Have Back Pain?

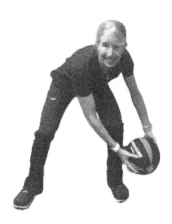

Many people have seen astronauts being carried on stretchers after months in space. It is not the trauma of launching a person into space that produces lumbar injuries. Specific changes occur in the body without a weight bearing stimulus for months. Most people know about decreased bone density and muscle mass, but did you know antigravity increases disc herniations in the lower back? Several studies have shown 52-70% of astronauts experience lower back pain, and it isn't necessarily from the trauma.

An article published in 2018 in *Spine Journal* examined how decreased gravity affected the lower back muscles. In the article titled "From the International Space Station to the Clinic: How Prolonged Unloading May Disrupt Lumbar Spine Stability," astronauts were evaluated before and after six months on the International Space Station.
https://www.ncbi.nlm.nih.gov/pubmed/28962911

The study found that the lumbar spine curve decreased by 11%, and active lumbar range of motion decreased over 20%. The water inside the lumbar disc did not change from before to after time in space; however, multifidus muscle mass decreased by 20%. As multifidus muscle mass decreased, there was an increased loss of lumbar curvature. Furthermore, those astronauts with severe lumbar degenerative changes presented with post-trip lumbar pain or disc herniations.

While most of us won't travel to the International Space Station, lumbar pain is associated with multifidus muscle loss, lumbar curvature loss, increased stiffness, and poor muscular stability.

A 2019 *Spine* study by Dr. Burkhart, "Negative Effects of Long Duration Spaceflight on Paraspinal Muscle Morphology," evaluated muscle mass changes in astronauts after long duration flights." https://www.ncbi.nlm.nih.gov/pubmed/30624302

The study found decreased muscle mass (5-8%) in the erector spinae, multifidus, quadratus lumborum (QL), and psoas muscles upon astronauts returning to earth. The erector spinae and multifidus muscles returned to previous levels after one year with recovery training. However the quadratus lumborum and psoas muscles continued to show decreased muscle mass levels two to four years post trip.

The body does not always make a lot of sense. Why would some muscles return to previous levels while others don't recover? How transferable is this to the general population? After strength and muscle mass loss caused by lower back pain, are the quadratus lumborum and psoas muscles slow to return to previous levels? Is the lumbar spinal curvature flattening associated with zero gravity or the quadratus lumborum and psoas muscle loss? Do patients with lower lumbar pain experience the slow return of psoas and quadratus muscle similar to astronauts?

We see many of these same signs and symptoms with patients who experience chronic lower back pain. Pain and injuries "shut down" many lower back muscles leading to atrophy and neuromuscular coordination dysfunction. Strength and endurance in some muscles do not return to previous levels without specific exercises (quadratus lumborum and psoas muscles). Without specifically targeting the deep spinal stabilizers (multifidus and transverse abdominis), most people do not directly engage the muscles and lose spinal stabilization, leading to future injuries.

Chapter 6: Treatment Philosophy

Treatment Philosophy 101: Slowly Bring a Bigger Hammer

I developed one of my treatment philosophies from Jeff, who I worked for at a golf course in my early college years (I have a lot of stories from Jeff and only a few can be written). Jeff had a tremendous talent for repairing and fixing equipment, everything from heavy construction equipment to expensive golf course mowers. He was able to troubleshoot and solve problems.

As you can imagine some equipment required precision and very gentle care, while other equipment required brute force.

Before I tell this story let me remind you I was 19 years old, so the left side of my brain wasn't exactly connected to the right side. I was on a very expensive greens mower, that was exceptionally fragile. Great care should be taken with the mowing reels that cut the greens heights to a few millimeters.

Lets say the last thing a dumb kid should do is to take a short cut with the mower and risk hitting the reel on a concrete golf course path. A horrible bang let me know metal was bent. I was freaking out that I destroyed the reel and would require many hours to fix. When you're making $5.50 an hour, a several thousand dollar reel is a month's worth of work.

I drove the mower to the shop. When Jeff saw me he knew two things: one was that I should not be back at the shop for a few hours. Second, the scared look on my face meant I broke something.

He examined the damage and walked back into the shop. He returned with a crowbar and three different sizes of sledgehammers. Initially I was unsure if the sledge hammers were for me or the mower.

He set the crow bar into position and grabbed the smallest hammer. He hit the bar with a tiny tap, larger tap, and then bigger tap. When that didn't produce the results, he grabbed the next bigger hammer. Same process with a tiny tap, bigger tap, and then even harder tap. Finally with the largest sledge hammer bent the reel casing back to the proper position.

After a few extra taps he looked up at me and said, "I've had a really bad day, so don't break anything else this week dumbA**; or you will be picking rocks for a month. And bring doughnuts tomorrow"

With great care and better judgment I worked all week without an additional incident. I had a significant amount of time to evaluate the situation. I broke the rule of never taking the greens mower across the sidewalk because I didn't understand it. Now I knew why the procedure was in place.

I also didn't know how to assess the damage. I was worried about the expensive mower parts and thought fixing them would require hours of grinding and sharpening the chipped reel. If I were in charge, I would have taken the wrong steps to correct the problem. I did not recognize the big picture, that I had luckily only damaged the steel protective case. So I had shown a lack of judgment and understanding of the problem.

It took me several hours to figure out why he brought three hammers to the mower. Jeff was not known for being subtle, gentle, or politically correct.

It took me a while to realize he was using extra caution. The largest hammer with a strong swing would definitely bend the metal, but it could be way too much and cause additional damage. Instead, Jeff started out more gently than he thought was required, just to make sure he wouldn't make the damage worse. He slowly increased the stimulus to create a reasonable response without causing more damage.

Treating Low Back Pain With Progressively Bigger Hammers

Treatment for chronic low back injuries needs to follow the same protocol. Start more gently than you think is necessary to make sure it doesn't flare up the problem. Then slowly increase the stimulus and challenge to create a reasonable response, and then push as hard as possible without creating a bigger problem.

The worst thing a provider can do is flare up a person by swinging a hammer that is too big on the first day. Day one should be about assessing the damage and creating a plan. Try a simple treatment that carries a low risk without making the situation worse. If day one goes well, then bring a greater stimulus for day two. Slowly increase the stimulus until meeting the threshold needed to fix the problem.

On day one, I want to see how your back responds to basic treatments. If all goes well I will add more on day two, and then even more on day three. If the little hammer makes you worse, then thankfully I did not hit you with a medium size hammer and really make you miserable. After understanding your problem, I can make better decisions on how hard to challenge you and the injury to create improvement with minimal risk of aggravation.

Jeff taught me a valuable lesson that day. I wish I could say that I have never pushed or exacerbated a patient's condition by being too aggressive. Sorry, sometimes I'm a slow learner.

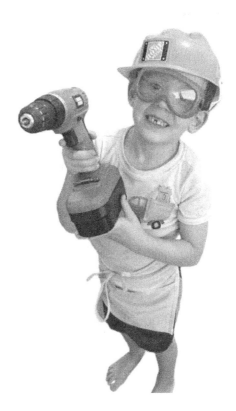

But I'd like to think we don't make those mistakes anymore, by being too aggressive early in treatment.

Side note:
I also do not want to give you the impression that Jeff only made great decisions. There is a story in which he became tired of weed eaters breaking in the creek full of cattails. His solution was to hand cut steel blades, creating a very indestructible cutting apparatus. Unfortunately his blades were not balanced, causing excessive vibration during operation, and making them was an OSHA violation. However, this was Montana in an era where safety features and OSHA were mostly optional.

Treatment Philosophy 102: No Treatment Plan Is Perfect

Low back pain is complicated because of the stresses, forces, postures, movements, muscles, and number of injured tissues. There are principles to a low back treatment plan. However, there is not a single plan to get everyone better. Multiple treatments work best for different people.

Research journals are full of studies about treatments that helped decrease pain and improve function. Flexion exercises versus extension exercises, acupuncture, massage, manual therapy, decompression, passive modalities combined with active exercises, chiropractic versus physical therapy, or different types of chiropractic adjustments all showed overall improvement.

The principles are the same for everyone, but the application of treatments and procedures are different for each person's recovery.

If there is one thing I hope you learn from this book (and I hope there is more than one), it is that there are treatments and procedures that will help decrease any person's pain and enhance daily function.

If a person is not improving from one treatment, I believe it is important to switch treatments. A different order or combination of treatments might be the key to getting a person past the recovery plateau.

A great clinic has a process and procedure to try multiple treatments. Bad clinics are "one trick ponies"; they only have one treatment for low back pain.

This week we had a patient come into our clinic with severe low back and sciatic pain. He had been suffering for a couple months. Physical therapy was not working at another clinic, and he described minimal improvement over the last eight weeks of treatment. A few minutes into the examination it became clear the other clinic was utilizing a very basic treatment plan for sprains.

He obviously had a disc injury, but the other provider was stuck on sprain treatments, explaining his lack of progress. The therapist told him to get surgery because therapy wouldn't help him.

Thankfully, he was questioning his therapist's skills and sought our office for a second opinion. The therapist was a one trick pony.

As you can imagine, the patient is getting better with lumbar disc treatments. He does have a difficult road ahead of him, but he has all the signs of improving and returning to pre-injury status without surgery.

This patient is a perfect example of why treatments should change based on progress or lack of improvement. He could have presented as a severe sprain the first few weeks, so I do not mean to throw the other provider under the bus; but the clinical picture I saw when he walked into our office was a disc herniation. The plan should have shifted or changed because of the lack of progress. Likewise, just because therapy did not work at that clinic, doesn't mean that a patient will not improve somewhere else.

We can help a lot of people, but sometimes a patient requires treatment at another clinic to improve to the next level. We won't help everyone, but we will definitely help many more than the "one trick pony" providers.

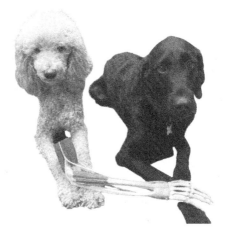

I absolutely encourage patients to research other treatment options, ask questions, and be active participants in their healthcare. If he hadn't searched out another option, the above patient would have gotten surgery that he didn't need, and that wouldn't have solved his problems.

Treatment Is a Progression
Initial treatment goals include:
- Getting you out of pain
- Increasing flexibility
- Restoring proper range of motion
- Increasing strength and endurance
- Restoring muscle coordination
- Restoring muscle stability around the back
- Restoring function and muscular stability around the feet, ankles, knees, hips, and back's neuromuscular systems

Treatment Philosophy 103: Providers & Chefs

McDonalds vs. Flemings
Sometimes a person needs a quick lunch and anything will work. A simple cheeseburger prepared quickly and consistently makes a billion people happy and serves a purpose. Expectations are different when going to a high end steak house such as Flemmings. Patrons expect different levels of quality and service, and the end product is very different.

Clinics Are Very Similar to Restaurants
Most clinics are somewhere in between McDonalds and Flemings, offering a variety of options for a reasonable price. Everybody has friendly staff. Some restaurants have better systems and cooks than others. Some places do a pretty good job with a big menu, while others do a really great job on a few dishes. With dinner you put in some effort finding a location that better fits your needs and purpose, and often spend more time researching restaurants than therapy clinics.

The Cook Is More Important than the Door Sign
Colorful and pretty signs might make you feel warm and fuzzy about the restaurant, but the true value is the cook's skill and ability. You can always tell when an average cook is just following a recipe. A better cook adjusts the seasoning as needed.

A great cook evaluates what ingredients he can put his hands on combining creativity and past experience. He relies on his team of cooks, waiters, and waitresses to give his patrons the best possible experience.

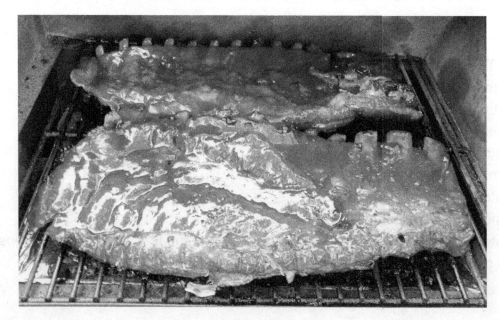

Treatment Philosophy 104: Look for Great Providers in Good Systems

Rehab should be about utilizing all of the tools and therapeutic concepts available to get you better. No single speciality or philosophy will solve every problem.

In many ways, it is less about the type of degree a person has and more about the provider's ability to use his or her "tool box" and problem solving skills. The initial examination and assessment determines the correct plan and first step. However, the plan should be flexible, based on your improvement and response to treatments. This is where the provider's skill and experience make the difference. A good provider modifies the treatment plant to achieve the best outcome.

A great provider is not afraid to admit that the plan is not working, and come up with a new plan.

Experience Counts

I worked with a physical therapist who was as experienced as Santa Claus, mainly because they went to kindergarten together (I stole that line from him). Eric had worked and done a lot of things in his career. He also had an incredible ability to motivate a patient into doing two or three exercises that provided the "greatest bang for their buck," including patients who vowed not to exercise at home.

He used his grey hair and storytelling to his advantage. Eric had a lot of stories and was really fun to work with. He was great at teaching difficult patients why and what they should be doing, and keeping it simple. He was also great at getting patients to build a solid foundation, and helping them to master an exercise before moving onto the next.

Too many times we hear patient stories about going to a therapist who "overshoots" and has a patient doing higher level activities than what he or she is ready to handle. This sets a patient up for failure.

Eric would make a joke about, "Kids these days. Back when I first started I would give a patient every exercise I knew. Fifteen minutes later, I would ice him down. Today's new graduates have a 70-year-old standing on one foot, pointing north, rubbing his belly, patting the top of the head, belly breathing, and focusing on proper stomach contractions."

The inexperienced new therapists all want to start with "new and cool exercises," even with a patient who can't perform the most basic foundation exercise.

"The kids" have not learned the importance of properly assessing a patient's functional ability and then providing slightly challenging exercises to move toward the end goal. Overshooting a patient's ability is always a disaster. In any skill, a person has to master the fundamentals first. If you can't hit a ball off a tee why try hitting a 100 mile-an-hour fastball?

Fun Fact: Professional baseball players spend more time practicing their form and improving their mechanics by hitting off a tee than younger players. At a batting cage a professional works on their mechanics by hitting off a tee. Meanwhile, most younger players skip the tee and swing at live pitches. The hitter that needs to improve his mechanics the most is least likely to hit off a tee.

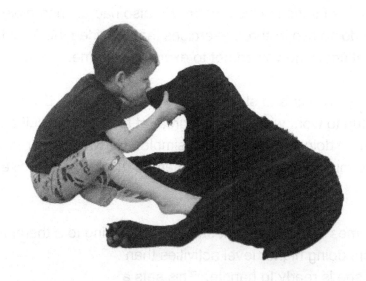

Treatment Philosophy 105:
Find The Right Provider, Even If You Have to Fire the Current One!

I hope you like the person you are working with. You should not have to work with someone you hate spending a few hours a week with. Unfortunately, being a pleasant and good person doesn't make him or her good at a job.

My dentist has a saying, "Patients only know if they like their dentist. They expect each visit to be a little unpleasant. The only person who knows how good your dentist was, is the next dentist looking in your mouth."

I hope you only meet good and likable people in every chiropractic and physical therapy clinic. Your provider needs to care about you and improve your quality of life, and he or she needs to work hard to do what's best for you.

My chiropractor growing up once said, "I get hired and fired every day, which takes some getting used to. Whether they liked me is not as important as that they know I did my best and worked hard to get them better every day."

As providers, we want to do our best for every patient, but sometimes a different provider and clinic can do a better job on this particular problem. We all can't be great at everything. If I can't get your back better, I hope you find a place that can provide the right services at the right time to solve your problem. Obviously the next provider won't be as fun or interesting as us, but I hope you get better. So fire me and hire the person who can get you better.

Side Note: When you are not fun or interesting, you need to distract patients with dogs begging for treats. That's why I always keep at least one dog in the office at all times.

When people ask me who works on my injuries, I tell them the truth. It depends on the problem. When I need only a spinal adjustment, there are a handful of people. When I need flexion distraction, I see one specific person. When I need Graston and soft tissue work, I see two people. Yes, I cherry pick. I have an understanding of what needs to be done and who has really good skills.

I see patients do the same thing in my office. They often request to work with someone for a specific activity, or they ask for a specific provider for an adjustment. Great! When patients can identify what works for them it enhances their therapy. It does not hurt our feelings - we are happy you are getting better.

Important Principles in Therapy

Identify the Weak Link

Over years people develop compensation mechanisms to protect the weak spot in their chronic low back pain. Muscle guarding, altered positions, and utilizing other muscles to protect the back are common examples.

Everyone has heard the phrase, "The weakest link in the chain breaks first." This is particularly true in the body.

The body wants to protect the weak link, and will sacrifice healthier tissue to reduce risk of injury.

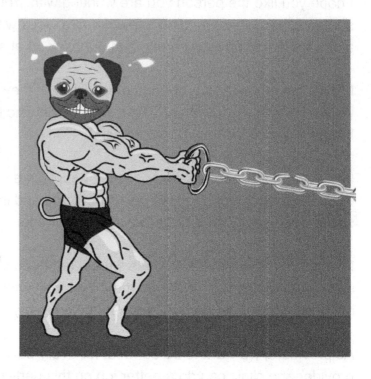

Unfortunately, with activity and strain, the weak spot always breaks first. This is why people describe their pain as always starting in the same spot, and progressing in a predictable pattern. A mild aggravation acts one way, and a moderate aggravation radiates further down the leg. A severe aggravation causes different symptoms.

The weak spot is a chronic condition that continues to deteriorate over time without proper intervention. The key is working on the weak spot in the kinetic chain and preventing future injuries.

Video: Why You Keep Getting Hurt: Stress Loads on Tissues

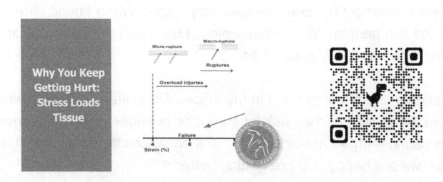

Pain vs. Function

Pain is a warning sign, much like the oil light in your car. The light does not tell you if the engine is working properly or optimally. The light will tell you when the oil is really low, but not when it is slightly low.

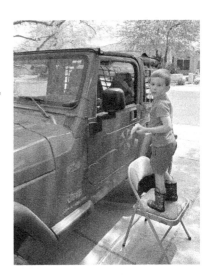

People do not depend on the oil light for determining the efficiency of the engine. However, people try to use pain to determine how the body is functioning. *Pain does not measure function.* Pain sensors activate when tissue is damaged enough to "turn on the light."

Pain sensors are not a measuring function!

Can't Wait for the Check Oil Light

My Grandpa would tell a story about my dad and his car maintenance. My grandpa was handy around the house and with cars, my dad was great at washing cars. Grandpa would say that my dad would wash his car every weekend and it was always clean, but would never open the hood. Why check the oil when the rims are clean? As you can imagine one day the clean car started smoking.

Waiting for the red warning light is a bad way to manage your favorite asset. Your back health should be checked just like the oil: it should be measured and checked *frequently*.

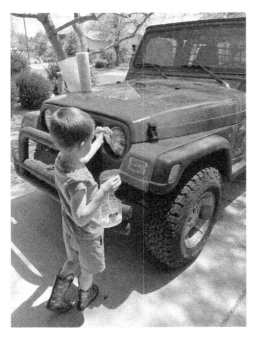

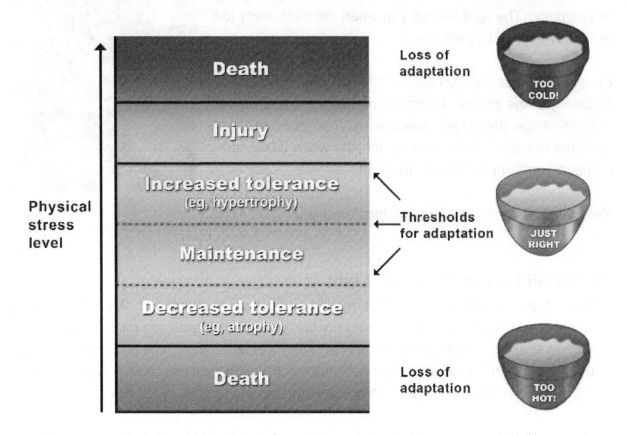

Goldy Locks and the Three Bears

Does your lower back feel better after walking for a while? Is it worse with too much sitting? Movement is usually good. However, it is similar to little Goldy Locks and her porridge: exercise can be too much, too little, or just right. The wrong amount will lead to a flare up. Just right will propel you further along toward your goals.

With too little exercise your back is overloading joints and ligaments, producing strain and pain on the tissue. With too much movement you are creating damage to other tissue. The right amount of activity leads to increased strength and feeling better.

"Too little, too much, or just right" is a theme throughout rehabilitation and therapy; the correct balance changes with progress and treatment needs to adjust to these changes.

Changes in Low Back Muscles with Chronic Pain

A 2017 study published in *Spine* looked at the integrity differences among lumbar muscles in patients with recurrent and chronic low back pain. The article titled, "Lumbar Muscle Structure and Function in Chronic Versus Recurrent Low Back Pain: a Cross Sectional Study" looked at lean muscle fat and activity of the multifidus and erector spinae during back extension. https://www.ncbi.nlm.nih.gov/pubmed/28456669

The study built off information from other studies showing that muscle atrophy, fat infiltration into muscle, changes in muscle fiber type, altered activity, and changes to biomechanics occurred in people with chronic low back pain. It utilized MRIs to analyze changes in muscle composition versus function. The study separated patients with recurrent low back pain from those with constant chronic low back pain.

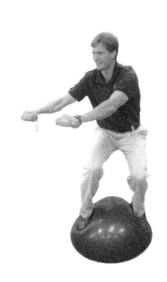

Chronic low back pain patients had increased fat infiltrate into the muscle and increased muscle hypertonicity (contraction) compared to the recurrent group. The structure and function of the muscle was different in people who suffered with constant back pain compared to those with episodes of pain.

Stabilization Exercises

A 2004 study published in *Spine Journal* demonstrated that hip stabilization was also compromised in patients with chronic low back pain. In the study, "Hip Strategy for Balance Control in Quiet Standing is Reduced in People with Low Back Pain;" individuals with chronic low back pain were four times more likely to fail testing for through lack of postural stabilization and core stability.
https://www.ncbi.nlm.nih.gov/pubmed/15014284

Although core muscle weakness is one of the problems leading to low back pain, glute weakness also contributes. Overactive hamstrings and hip flexors attempt to stabilize the pelvis and lumbar spine. Exercises that activate, engage, and coordinate the glute muscles with the core are necessary for long term improvement.

Exercises that optimize glute function help stop the hamstrings from over engaging to create pelvic stability. Please do not dust off the 1980s VHS of "Buns of Steel." Instead, focus on therapeutic exercises to avoid aggravating the lower back.

Spinal stabilization is very important to eliminate lower back pain. The spinal joints are one piece of the puzzle, all joints in the spine, pelvis, and lower extremity require proper stabilization to enhance function and prevent injuries.

Video: <u>Gait Theory of Pain</u>

Rusty Door Hinge Theory

The rusty door hinge is my personal phrase for explaining stuck and sore joints. We are all familiar with a rusty door hinge that locks up and prevents movement. It takes a fair amount of work rocking the rusty hinge to restore movement and break the rust.

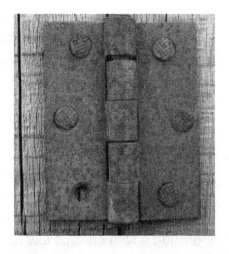

Spinal joints follow this principle when injured; they lock up and do not move when injured. The body tries to protect injuries by limiting motion and movement. The body thinks if it doesn't let you keep moving then you can't keep hurting it. Unfortunately, locking up joints actually causes more pain.

Joints have movement and pain sensors inside them. Decreased signals from movement sensors combined with increased pain signals leads to pain and muscle spasms. Unfortunately muscle spasms further compress injured joints, producing increased pain sensation, and additional muscle spasms further limit joint motion.

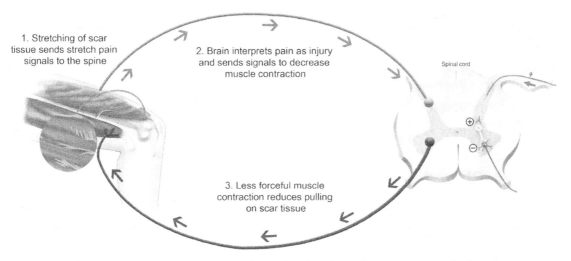

Eliminating scar tissue stops the pain signals and restores muscle function.

A cycle develops of increased pain signals causing muscle spasms, limiting joint movement, and producing increasing joint sensor pain and muscle spasms. The cycle continues until movement is restored in joints and the brain receives signals saying "everything is okay."

Treatment has to break the chronic pain cycle and restore motion; disrupting the pain feedback loop from all sources of pain. Rust inside the door hinges needs to be broken up, allowing for proper motion and movement. It's not as easy as adding WD-40 to restore motion - we have to do it the hard way.

"How do you want to play the game?"

There are infinite possibilities for treating your lower back pain. We can be more aggressive in treatment frequency, variety of modalities, advanced imaging, number of exercises, or challenge. We can utilize pain management physicians for epidural or facet injections, or prescribe oral medication and topical creams.

There are numerous combinations; however, treatment needs to consider goals, timeline, work schedule, home commitments, and ability to spend time working on your condition.

I ask a patient what his/her goals, timeline, schedule, and expectations are to give that person treatment options that meet the objectives. If a person requires significant improvement fast because he is leaving on a European tour in two weeks, treatment recommendations will include immediate referrals to pain management. If he would prefer avoiding an MRI and time is on his side, we can delay advanced imaging for a few weeks and see how he responds to conservative treatment.

In a sense, treatment is similar to choosing your own adventure book. We can modify a treatment plan based on many factors, especially your functional goals and time frame.

Chess vs. Chutes & Ladders

Treatment plans and decision making are similar to playing chess: making strategic moves with a plan after evaluating the board. We want to make good decisions for the best possible outcomes. We never want to treat your healthcare like a game of Chutes & Ladders, where we randomly move across the board with frequent setbacks.

Furthermore, poor patient decisions increase the odds of setbacks.

If cleaning the house flares up the lower back for three days, then the patient needs to stop cleaning the house until he or she is ready to handle the workload. Live with a messy house or get someone else to do it. Eventually a person can perform small increments of cleaning without pain.

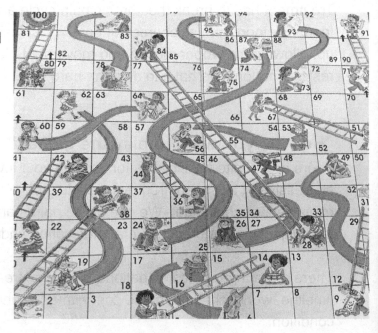

Activities that really aggravate the lower back, such as scrubbing tubs and vacuuming, can wait until there is significant improvement.

Increasing the workload on the lower back without a strategy is playing Chutes & Ladders. Assessing functional levels and workload, and increasing at a reasonable rate is playing chess. **Be reasonable!**

Some Is Good More Is *Not* Better

In the early stages of rehab, pushing your limits and doing too much is always bad. It never works out for the patient. Challenging broken tissue causes *more tissue damage*, not a miraculous recovery.

There are smart patients who learn this lesson after the first trial and some take a couple of trials. The really stubborn ones have the most flare ups and are always disappointed with their progress. These individuals always ask: "Why am I not getting better?" I respond with: "Because you don't learn and keep doing dumb s***!"

Close Only Counts with Horseshoes, Hand Grenades and Slow Dancing

This statement doesn't need an explanation.

Treatment & Exercises Can Be Like Watering Your Lawn

With very little water, grass does not grow, and you have a barren dirt patch. Too much water floods the grass and slows growth. A just-about-right amount produces a great lawn.

Successful treatment requires a similar type of balance

Just Because You Can Doesn't Mean You Should

If only I had learned to appreciate this phrase in my 20s, life would have been much easier. Pushing your lower back through an activity it is not accustomed to usually leads to a flare up. Just because you can pick up a 60-inch TV and carry it upstairs, doesn't mean your back won't regret it. Just because you want to lift weights doesn't mean your back ligaments are ready to handle the stress load. Just because your floors are dirty and you want them mopped doesn't mean your body won't punish you tomorrow morning.

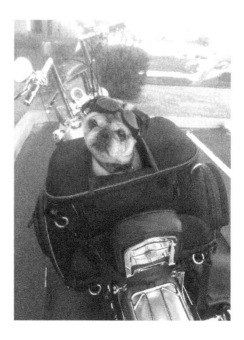

Mom's Legendary Cookies

When I was a college freshman living in the dorm, my mom sent homemade cookies. Baked goods are usually more valuable than money or beer in a freshman dorm; however, this box of cookies was false advertising.

The chocolate cookies looked normal. Maybe a little hard and burned, but that was her trademark. These, however, also had a bite that can only be described as the recipe called for two teaspoons of salt but was replaced with two cups. They were bad, but they soon became legendary.

My roommate Charlie and I had a dilemma. We did not want to eat them, but felt bad throwing them away. Our resident advisor Kelly came down the hall and was saying hi. Charlie very smoothly offered the bag to Kelly saying we had extra. Once again, cookies in a dorm are like gold and he happily went down the hall.

Five minutes later he shows back up at our door, very politely explaining he appreciates the cookies but he does not need that many and gives the bag back. We were unsuccessful in trying to pass the bag to other residents. You can imagine how bad the chocolate cookies had to be that no one in a dorm would eat them.

She cared enough to make and send cookies, but execution was missing. There are a lot of chocolate chip recipes. Some are fantastic, most will be good enough, some are bad, and some are legendary dorm bad.

This is the same problem with clinics and treatment plans. Some clinics are outstanding and others are good. Some look good from six feet away, but the substance and execution are lacking. It does not matter how high tech the office, amount of expensive equipment, or if they take your insurance. At the end of the day, the product is what matters. Did you get better and lay the groundwork for preventing future injuries?

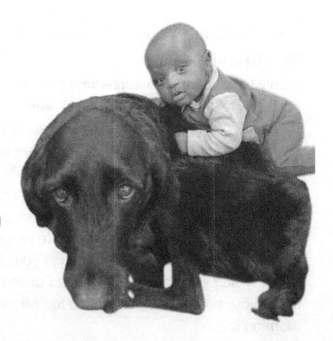

Mountain Climbers Scaling a Vertical Cliff

Treatment needs to identify all of the weak links in your movement patterns and properly restore stability and neuromuscular control to the system. Therapy will provide better ways of tracking your function than pain. Restoring joint motion and muscle mass enables spinal stabilizers and the brain to better control the vertebrae and reduce excessive joint strain. Therapy guides your decision making and teaches you to be reasonable in your activities, finding the "just right" amount of sitting, standing, bending, walking, twisting, and driving.

One of the keys to successful treatment is to keep it simple and focus on what's important.

Picture five mountain climbers scaling a vertical cliff, all tied to the same rope. The climbers work together to move toward the top. The top climber can't leave the group behind, and the bottom climber can't pass the climbers above him. If the bottom two climbers are not progressing then the whole group stays on the cliff. All the climbers need to move in a coordinated sequence for the group to reach the top.

The bottom climber determines the risk of injury. Even if the other team members are strong, the bottom climber can pull the group back down the cliff if he isn't capable of ascending it.

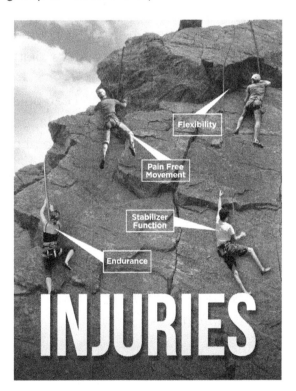

In therapy, these climbers from top down correspond to range of motion, flexibility, strength, endurance, and joint stability. Treatment gets all of the climbers to the top of the mountain. If treatment only focuses on flexibility and strength improvement, the group stops making progress when endurance and stability stop improving. You can't reach full therapeutic goals unless all aspects of function improve.

Usually when people present with a chronic problem, their past attempts at treatment have failed to stabilize the joints. Even with everything else improving, risk of future injuries remains with unstable joints. All of the goals are important.

Dr. Google

I am a firm believer in learning, hence the book. However, learning facts and parts of the puzzle creates problems. I'm sure I can find a YouTube channel on brain surgery, a *Brain Surgery For Dummies* on Amazon, and a neighbor who knows all about it. With this combined information I should be ready to perform surgery, right?

Facts and information are easy to come by in today's age. The application of treatment and therapies is difficult to find and even harder to apply correctly.

A patient came into the office this week with a severe case of medial epicondylitis, or golfer's elbow. He was an avid racquetball player and then stopped for over a year. He was playing pickleball the last few months, but it is a very different activity for the forearms compared to racquetball.

He decided to start playing racquetball again, and very quickly developed elbow pain. A few Google searches led him to his diagnosis of medial epicondylitis, which was correct. A couple more clicks led him to a golfer's elbow support, which he was wearing incorrectly. A couple of YouTube videos provided exercises to eliminate his pain. The exercises are great, and will help him in four weeks when he improves 50%. Right now the exercises are just making his injury worse.

Dr. Google is a resource, and can be a great way to learn and educate. It is not a very good tool for determining injury stages and giving step by step treatment progressions for your injury. Using the example above of mountain climbers,

Google treatment plans tend to emphasize only one or two mountain climbers and the rest are ignored or pushed off the cliff.

Read a good book on low back pain to get a better understanding of chronic injuries and treatments.

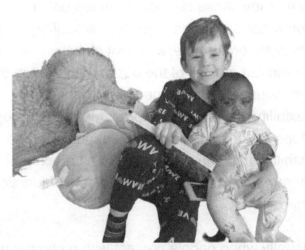

Chapter 7: Spinal Stabilization -Working On The System

What Are the Best Treatments?
The treatment that improves your weakest spots and reduces the risk of future pain is the best treatment for you. There are many types of compensation mechanisms, and finding ways to stabilize the weakest link is the most important. The best treatments are the "right combinations of exercise, at the right time, in the right order."

What Does Core Strengthening Mean?
When a person has chronic low back pain and multiple levels of disc herniations, I compare their low back to a jenga set. The spinal joints are wobbly and uncontrolled, and excessive motion occurs all over the place. Core strengthening is about teaching all of the muscles to work together again, and properly stabilize and protect the lower back discs and joints.

Think of juggling. You can have the strength to juggle and still drop the balls. Juggling is more about coordination of movement to keep five balls flying through the air. People with chronic low back pain tend to have horrible juggling skills, and our job is to teach you how to toss one ball in the air properly and then two, three, four, and finally five.

Video:
Stability and Risk Factors

How Do I Strengthen My Core?

The short answer is not the way you think: crunches and sit ups are not helpful. Exercise classes can be if you get lucky. If you have enough juggling skills when you walk into an exercise class, and it happens to strengthen your weak spots, then you will improve. Otherwise, the exercise class might flare up your back rather than making it better.

Just as with juggling, a series of fundamental steps and exercises need to take place in the proper order to get you from uncoordinated to impressive. Trying to skip steps always leads to failure.

In the office a very good high school running back had been working at increasing his core and hip stability because he was lacking in these areas, leading to former injuries. He was working hard in weight training and at practice, but the exercises were not targeting the correct muscle groups well enough.

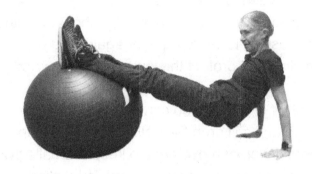

Our exercise specialist, Nina, was working with him on a difficult core routine. She volunteered to do a few sets with him for support, and she absolutely destroyed him. He could not keep up with her; and learned the hard way that young and strong does not mean anything in core stability. I just watched and drank my coffee, because I am smart enough to know the series was going to hurt.

She would kill me if I printed her age, but let's say she is closer to the football player's grandmother's age than mother's. Nina has done an incredible job of working on her core strength and stability, and definitely does not have back pain. Despite his core weakness, the player is an incredible athlete, and I can't wait to see what happens with him when his core strength improves to match the rest of his athleticism.

Proper Neuromuscular Control

A 2018 study published the *Journal of International Neuromodulation Society* discusses the role of multifidus and transverse abdominis weakness in patients with chronic low back pain. Weakness in these muscles increases pain perception in the vertebral joints due to functional instability of the lumbar spine. The authors of "Muscle Control and Non Specific Back Pain" suggest that targeting the lower back muscles and increasing neurostimulation can overcome the negative pain signals that effectively shut down proper spinal joint control. https://www.ncbi.nlm.nih.gov/pmc/articles/PMC5814909/

How Should Your Body Control Spinal Movements?

Spinal joint movement should be controlled by the deep spinal and deep core muscles. With chronic pain, these muscles get "shut off" and the superficial (outside) muscles attempt to control spinal movements.

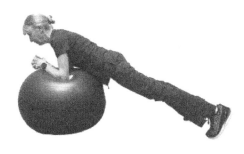

Posture throughout the day is significantly compromised by lack of deep muscle activity and overuse of the superficial muscles. A 2005 study published in the *Clinical Journal of Pain* examined these muscle activation changes. Significant muscle neuromuscular dysfunction was found in the study titled, "Are the Changes in Postural Control Associated with Low Back Pain Caused by Pain Interference?"

In the study, researchers found decreased transverse abdominis and obliquus internus activation and increased activation of obliquus externus to maintain postural stability in patients with chronic low back pain. Pain led to the improper use of muscles to control spinal movements.

Compensatory use of superficial muscles leads to inefficient movements and increased joint pain. When facet joints and ligaments send pain signals to the brain, the body responds by over-activating specific muscles for stabilization. These muscles are inefficient, and often lead to those big injuries that occur when bending down to pick up a shoe up or pet the dog.

Posture and Movement Stability Use the Same Mechanisms

Because posture and movement utilize the same neural mechanisms and pathways for stability, failure in one system comprises the other.

For example, if a person has difficulty maintaining postural stability, he or she will likely have difficulty maintaining joint stability during movement.

A 2016 study published in *Advances in Experimental Medicine and Biology*, titled "The Relation Between Postural and Movement Stability," reported:

> As a consequence, the same stabilizing mechanisms, instead of resisting motion from the initial posture, drive the body to another stable posture. In other words by shifting spatial thresholds, the nervous system converts movement resisting movement-producing mechanisms. It is illustrated that, contrary to the conventional view, this control strategy allows the system to transfer body balance to produce locomotion and other actions without losing stability at any point of them. It also helps orient posture and movement with the direction of gravity. It is concluded that postural and movement stability is provided by a common mechanism.

Will Yoga / Pilates / Exercise Class / Trainer Fix My Core Issues?

If your weakness is just a little below the class level, these classes could be a perfect fit and engage your weak links in the kinetic chain. If that happens, the class is great for the individual. I have heard many stories about people starting an exercise routine and how it changed their life and back pain levels.

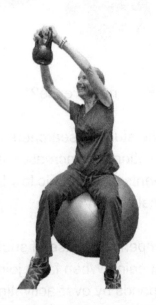

It does not always work out that way.

How Will a Person Know if the Class Isn't Helping?
You keep getting hurt. Although exercise makes you feel better, you will continue to experience back sprains and strains with activity. In the old days you would feel pain when sitting on an airplane for longer than an hour, and now it takes a five-hour flight to feel the same discomfort. Instead of experiencing back pain episodes six times a year, it only flares up twice a year.

Symptoms are better but a plateau has formed. Despite the level of exercise and activity, flare ups keep happening.

Great Example of Not Taking Proper Steps Forward

One of my favorite stories is about a woman who came into the office with severe lower back pain. Getting out of a chair was a monumental task and walking down the hallway looked painful. She was miserable. Apparently this happened every couple of months.

She had a history of chronic back pain and started going to Bikram yoga, which significantly improved her daily back pain. Her job required her to travel frequently. The day before she had returned from a 12-day trip of multiple hotel beds and flights. She had not had any sharp pain experienced in the last few days, but was noticing more tightness and stiffness in her back.

Since she was a little sore from traveling and had not been to a class for two weeks, she went to a yoga class that night. She described being stiff and worked at getting a great deep stretch in class. However she woke up in the middle of the night in severe and debilitating pain.

I tried to explain that her back was fatigued from the trip and probably a little guarded. The trip had overwhelmed her level of core strength and she had slightly aggravated it. The flight back or yoga pushed her back over the edge. Going to yoga was not a bad idea, but her back could not handle being pushed in its slightly aggravated state. She would have been better off taking it easy in class or performing a few light poses at home. The deep stretches she thought would provide relief actually aggravated her weak spot.

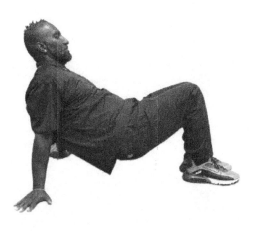

Hopefully her severe pain was her body overcompensating and guarding for a minor lumbosacral strain. The body remembers past episodes of severe injuries and is trying to protect itself against them. Basically, the body can overreact similar to a three-year-old being told "no." If things start to improve dramatically in a few days, that would be the root cause. However she could have also caused something bigger and we wouldn't know for a few days until her symptoms progressed or she got an MRI.

I went over the plan for acute rehab and that down-the-road therapy would include a few exercises to correct her core weakness and dysfunction in the kinetic chain. Right then she went on a tirade about how Bikram yoga was the greatest thing ever, and it fixed her back pain. Yoga could not cause her injury because it prevents back pain.

I think she would have liked to have stormed out of the office for dramatic effect, but she needed help getting out of the chair and down the hallway. She did not like my answer and did not reschedule for another appointment.

A few years later I opened the treatment room door and she was sitting in severe pain again. I recognized her immediately but she didn't recognize me or the office. She had filled out new patient paperwork and had a new last name. I let her tell her story of severe bouts of pain every couple of months that would last anywhere from one week to three. It occurred more often after traveling, especially longer trips. She went to Bikram yoga regularly and it had improved her back, in fact she had gone the previous night after getting home from a long trip. She felt really good afterwards but woke up in severe pain. She had seen a chiropractor for her back a few years ago but it didn't help.

I asked her if she felt like this was deja vu. Would she like to try my exercises this time, or come back in a few years in the same position? That's when it hit her.

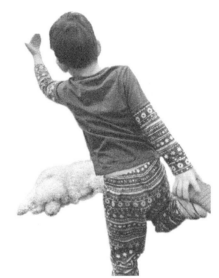

Just like the pyramids, when the foundation is built with cracks and weaknesses it will continue to crumble under sufficient stress. It can be as simple as changing a few activities and exercises to solidify the foundation. Regular Bikram yoga improved her quality of life, but she needed something a little different to fix her weak spots and move to the next level.

Picking Your Battles

With beginning exercise activity you have to be honest about your strength, endurance, and functional levels. Acting as if you are 25 again will definitely lead you to my office. Be honest about your physical activity. Acting like you are 90 when you're 40 is not good for anyone. Be realistic about your physical condition and what your body can handle.

Video:
Conrad and a Yard Full of Rock Story

My parents bought a house in the Sun Lakes retirement community and it needed some work. My dad called me on Friday and said that 13 tons of rock would be delivered that day. He asked if I could come help. I said, "You mean shovel 13 tons of rock while you supervise? No, I have to work today but I will be there tomorrow morning."

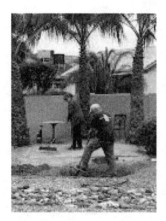

Since he makes bad decisions, my father decided to shovel the rock into a wheelbarrow and spread it through the yard by himself. The next morning when I got to his house there was a small pile of rocks in the driveway and a large old man laying on the tile floor.

Three weeks later he was still complaining about his back pain and all the rock he "*had to shovel.*" He is a great example of making bad decisions and not realistically assessing his physical condition. If he actually paid for treatment in my office, it would have cost him more in medical bills than hiring help or waiting 24 hours for super cheap labor (me).

Video: Bad Decisions #24: Old Man & The Hot Tub

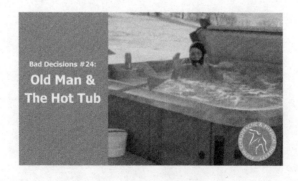

I Make Bad Decisions, and a Few Good Ones

At age 30, I dug an entire landscaping drip system by hand during an Arizona summer. At 40 I rented a trencher to dig the drip line and shoveled the dirt back in the trench by hand. When I am 50, all irrigation digging will be outsourced to someone else. I am not in the condition I was at 30, and I definitely will not be at 50. So at 66 if I decide to shovel 13 tons of rock and wheelbarrow it across the yard, I deserve to get hurt for making bad decisions.

Speaking of Bad Decisions

I was running a 100 mile race through the Arizona desert a few years ago. Yes, I did think about it before signing up and did a moderate amount of training beforehand. On race day I had a tremendous amount of respect for the distance and a fair amount of concern for the day's task. There is nothing like running for most of the day, realizing you have already run two marathons, and have two more to go.

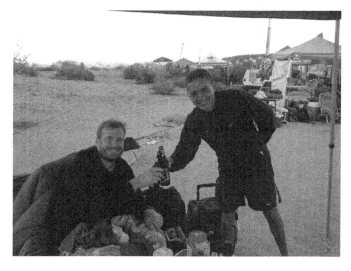

The race went as you might expect with a progressive slowdown as exhaustion set in. Race directors are wise enough to know runners make bad decisions after 75 miles, so a fresh escort can partner with the runner and hopefully make better decisions.

I had two friends who paced me through the end of the race. One friend was tremendous; he was positive and motivating. Arnie kept me going to the end. The other was helpful and embarrassing. If I'd had the energy, I would have shuffled off and left him in the desert to find his way back. My six-foot four-inch friend, CJ, showed up in exercise tights to "keep his calves warm."

It was cooler for the early morning hours, but it was not cold. CJ was the only runner in tights that night. We would meet up with other runners and they would taunt him on the trail. You know it must have been bad if a person who had run 80 miles could muster the energy to make fun of a person's wardrobe on Halloween weekend.

I do appreciate that CJ showed up and supported me for 15 miles through the desert at 2:00 a.m. Not many friends would do that.

Returning to the topic of bad decisions: I survived the 100-mile run without any significant injury, besides being really sore for a week. Of the two of us, only CJ ended up in the hospital that weekend. His appendix ruptured, and we might have seen signs of it toward the end of his loop. His wife believed that it was due to running 15 miles through a rocky trail while out of shape. I believe it was because his tights were too tight!

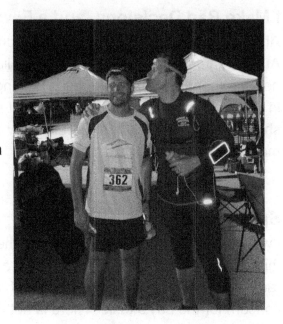

CJ and I have made a lot of bad decisions together over the years, and most will never end up in a book unless he runs for public office. His bad decision that weekend was posing for the picture, now that I have published it to the entire world. What are good friends for?

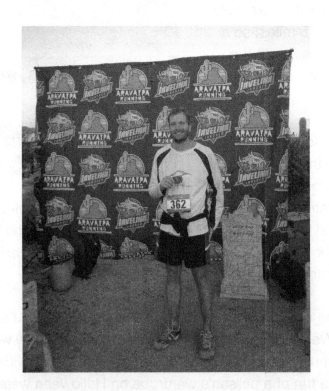

Chapter 8: Common Phrases From People Who Make Bad Decisions

My Pain For The Past 30 Years is Due To A Herniated Disc

People might have had their first extreme episode of low back pain 30 years ago from a herniated or extruded disc. However a disc does not stay herniated for 30 years. It will eventually patch itself back up in a year or two. Usually people begin to experience other types of back pain in the same region, leading to chronic low back pain and dysfunction.

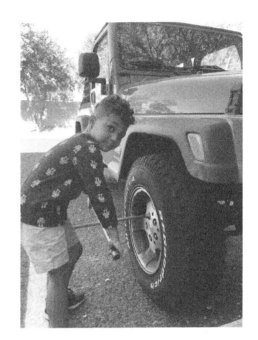

This Will Be Quick My Pain Started After..

Coughing, sneezing, vomiting, awkward lift, and excessive exercise all produce extreme intra-abdominal pressure and could result in a disc herniation. Some people develop disc injuries after a week of the flu: vomiting combined with several days of laying in bed. Not all injuries occur after lifting.

It Is Only a Little Worse - Constant, Burning, Aching, or Radiating to the Foot

All are not very good signs. Severe constant pain that radiates past the knee and into the foot is a sign of severe injuries. If the pain gets worse with coughing, sneezing and several orthopedic tests, it is usually caused by a lumbar disc injury.

My Back Is Killing Me, But It Is Not a Big Deal?

If the low back pain is similar to past episodes, then it is usually an aggravation of the weak link. If the pain is worse, different, or radiating further down the leg, my level of concern increases.

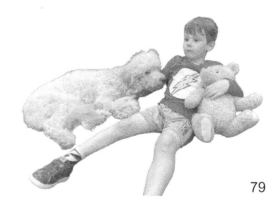

It Is Probably Just a Muscle Strain. Will It Go Away?
My favorite line from patients. If it was a muscle it wouldn't hurt for months, be severe, or radiate to your foot. It wouldn't be worse with movement, bending, twisting, or coughing. But if it makes you feel better to say it's a muscle...

I Just Pinched a Nerve...
Another myth that needs to be corrected. Nerve compression is a serious condition that results in loss of muscle strength, reflex, or sensation down the leg. Compression of a nerve can result in severe pain in a distinct pattern down the leg. A sharp shooting pain in the back is not a pinched nerve, thankfully.

But the Pain Radiates Down My Leg, Isn't That a Pinched Nerve?
Not necessarily. There are a lot of injuries that produce radiating pain. Referred or radiating pain can be caused by many types of injuries including central canal stenosis or neural foraminal nerve compression. Ligament sprains, muscle strains, joint capsule injuries, and nerve compression from muscle spasms can all produce radiating pain. Pain radiating down the leg does not mean a nerve is pinched.

Video: Can a Chiropractor Help with a Disc Bulge or Herniated Disc?

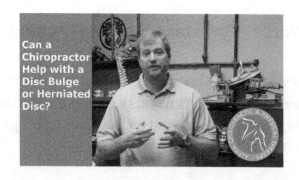

I Will Just Do Sit Ups to Get Stronger

Sit ups are one of the worst things you can do with a compromised lower back. A sit up places increased pressure on the front of the disc, causing forces to push backward on the disc. Disc herniations, bulges, and extrusions do not need anymore backward pressure.

Furthermore, sit ups are not the best exercise to strengthen the rectus abdominis muscle (think six pack of stomach). Anterior planks are much better, even modified planks from your knees are better. During the movement of a sit up, most people activate their psoas muscles (hip flexor) to pull the torso toward the legs.

Additionally, with chronic lower back pain the psoas muscle becomes shortened and hyperactive. Therapy is going to relax this muscle and decrease its activity. So why would you make rehab harder by doing sit ups?

Crunches are better at working the rectus abdominis. However, care has to be taken to maintain the lumbar arch and not overload the front of the discs. Exercises in the back of the book will show a crunch on a therapy ball. Be smart about this exercise.

Video:

<u>If You Can't Squat on One Foot Why Lift Heavy Weights?</u>

I Just Need One Good Crack…

This is like trying to swing for a home run on the first pitch: it is a strategy that does not work very well. Just as in baseball, the more successful teams get a lot of singles and doubles to score runs. A few home runs happen, but that is not the entire strategy.

I'm sure that strategy worked once, when you are a lot younger and with a mild joint

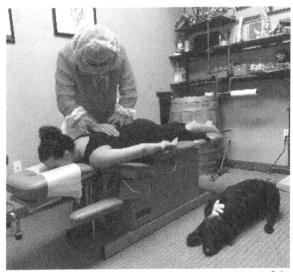

irritation, but not with a severe sprain, degenerated joints, or a disc injury.

Stupid YouTube Video Cracks…

Stupid and irresponsible things are posted online all the time. I have seen a few from chiropractors that make me cringe. I actually had a young guy come into the office and request a very high velocity adjustment to "really open everything up." He showed me the video, and it just looked stupid.

After explaining to him that I thought it was stupid, and it would probably hurt him, he asked, "so you're not going to do it?" All I could think of to say was "absolutely not."

Instead we did the appropriate type of adjustment for his pain and showed him some exercises for the long term. He wanted a home run type of adjustment instead of doing the work to fix his problems.

The next day his girlfriend gave the clinic a very low Google rating and claimed we didn't even adjust him. This was one of the days that goes with, "here is your sign."

Video:
A Patient Wanted His Money's Worth

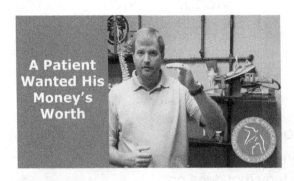

Chapter 9: Mistakes People Make

Exercises That Load Lumbar Discs

Sit ups, leg lifts, straight leg deadlifts, squats (when the chest hinges forward), leg press, and leg extensions on machines. My general rule is that if your high school PE teacher thought it was a great exercise, don't do it. Remember, he was working with a bunch of teenagers without back problems.

Video:

[Hinging at the Low Back Causes Pain](#)

Keep Doing What You're Doing

If your process was working, your back would be much stronger, flexible, and have great neuromuscular control. And you would not be reading this book. You need a different pathway to improve your back health.

Doing What Your Friends Do

This goes hand-in-hand with the previous paragraph. If your friends have chronic back pain, just smile and nod at their advice. If they have reached the functional exercises goals in this book then listen to how they did it, understanding your injury is probably different than theirs.

Years ago I had my dad do a series of exercises and stretches for his low back. He forgot them and at the next visit I showed him again. This went on for years. Finally we took a video of him doing the exercises properly.

Problem solved, right? On the next trip I asked how his back was feeling and about the exercises. He said, "I've been doing them every day but my back still hurts." I asked him to show me, and they were absolutely not the exercises I showed him. Those are for a completely different problem. At first he claimed they were the exercises I showed him until the video proved otherwise.

Video:
Conrad's and Fogerty Exercise Theories

He later admitted that he started doing his best friend's exercises because it helped his back pain, and they were easier. My dad grudgingly acknowledged that his friend still had daily back pain but it didn't hurt to golf anymore. If both of those guys would stop doing basic range of motion and progress to core stabilization they would be feeling better.

This is actually how the office videos and email started, in an attempt to not show my dad the same exercises for the 10th time. It did not work.

Not All Exercises Are Good for Everyone

Not everyone is equal. Everyone has different strength, endurance, flexibility, degenerated discs, arthritic joints, and wear and tear on their backs. It is silly to think everyone should start on the same exercises and progress at the same rate.

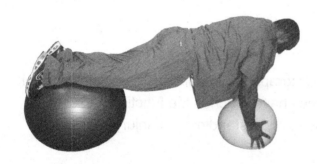

Certain exercises will be great for your friend, but will actually overload your weak spot. Likewise, the exercises could be strengthening your strong areas and not addressing your weakened muscles or poor spinal stabilization.

Building a strong back is similar to building the great pyramids of Giza; without a strong and solid foundation the pyramids would have crumbled.

The first set of exercises build the first layer of the foundation, and the next exercises build the second level. If you tried to perform fourth level exercises on a first-level foundation, injuries will result. Each level and layer has to be mastered before moving to the next level.

84

The biggest mistake people make is performing exercises that are too advanced. It might go well a few times, but sooner or later it will cause an injury.

Blaming Genetics - My Family Has a History Of Low Back Pain...

My response is, "My Grandpa John had a John Wayne Limp, does that mean I should have a limp? Of course he broke his leg crashing a race car and again falling off a roof."

Yes, genetic structure can play a role in bone development, body structure, and size. Most of us earn our back pain and injuries through activity in a lifetime. If your family members were all in construction, they would all have significant wear and tear injuries.

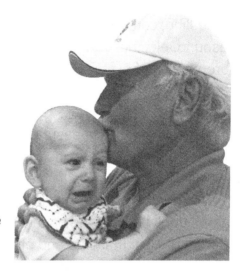

Years ago I had a patient try to blame his genetics for predisposing his shoulder and back pain. My response was, "or it could be related to your college football career followed by five years as a rodeo clown for bull riding."

It is easier to blame genetics than look at the history of wear and tear activities on the body.

Focusing on Pain Levels and Not Functional Goals

People are motivated by pain, and probably would only read this book after suffering from serious recurrent episodes of low back pain. A person's primary motivation in seeking treatment from chiropractors and physical therapists is to decrease pain. I have never had a patient come into the office saying that he or she felt great and wanted to enhance function to the highest level possible

Almost any treatment or exercise will help decrease pain levels from a flare up. I have seen many studies conclude that massage, acupuncture, chiropractic, physical therapy, dry needling, core exercises, stability training, running, yoga, tai chi, pilates, cold laser, ultrasound, electric, traction, spinal decompression, walking, stretching, and many different types of exercise classes decrease lower back pain for 4-12 weeks.
https://www.ncbi.nlm.nih.gov/pmc/articles/PMC6305160/pdf/jpr-12-095.pdf

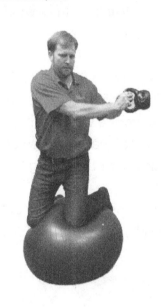

When the studies only measure pain for a short period of time, they often state that one treatment is effective. The treatment is effective at reducing pain for a couple months. However, if I was the patient would I want to go through treatment only to have the pain return in several months, or find out that all of that time and effort does not reduce the likelihood of future occurrences? Heck no: I would want efficient and effective treatments that would reduce my future injury risks.

Treatment has to reduce your pain, and then focus on improving lower back function. Great treatment also gives you a plan to continue and improve your spinal stability.

Video: <u>Spinal Stabilization from Tiny Stabilizers</u>

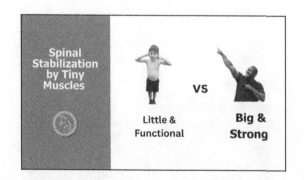

Chapter 10: Scapula & Mid Back

Having poor posture does not always mean that a person will have upper back or shoulder pain, but it does increase the likelihood. Upper cross syndrome causes elevation and shifting of the scapula, which changes the position of the glenohumeral joint: the joint in which the humerus (upper arm bone) inserts into the glenoid fossa (socket) at the shoulder. The altered position places extra stress on the rotator cuff muscles, and *all of the scapular stabilizer muscles.*

It also creates a weakened area in the mid back which produces a chronic dull ache and stiffness between the shoulder blades. Do you have "chronic knots" that you want someone to rub or work on frequently?

I think it makes sense to look at all of the muscles and tendons involved in shoulder movements and scapular stabilization. It's amazing how many times I see patients who have been treated for mid back or shoulder pain at other clinics and end up in my office with the same problem a year later.

As providers we can always decrease tendon pain with treatments, time, and rest. However, without removing the exacerbating stress underlying the problem, the injury is likely to return.

Elevated Shoulder Blades Are the First Falling Domino

Many injuries aren't spontaneous, particularly for older adults. Muscles and tendons show signs of degeneration prior to the individual experiencing pain. While a single event such as lifting improperly may exacerbate the injury, it is typically the final straw and not the root cause. A lifetime of improper movements and chronic poor posture created weakness, tissue injuries, and have been filling the "injury penny jar for years."

This book has likely made you more aware of the role the scapula (shoulder blades) play in movement. While most people aren't aware of the position of their shoulder blades, problems leading to neck and shoulder pain inevitably involve this area. Over time, the shoulder blades elevate and rotate, due to shortening of the upper trapezius, levator, pectoralis minor, and sternocleidomastoid muscles.

The lower trapezius, rhomboids, and serratus posterior muscles are placed in a less ideal position, and are eventually "shut off" or less active. They can't keep up in this altered scapular position. Scapula positional changes compromises cervical and thoracic joint stabilization, along with the glenohumeral joint.

Altered positions and movements lead to excessive tissue strain. Remember the shooting a cannon off a canoe example? When the scapular stabilizers can no longer do their job, the cannon is shooting off an unstable base. The canoe is moving all over the place.

For the scapula, that means that it is subtly shifting during arm movements, and not providing the concrete base for the arm to anchor its movements from. These subtle shifts are overloading other muscles and tendons as they try extra hard to hold the scapula still. With repetition, these less than ideal movements create soft tissue injuries that add up in wear-and-tear injuries.

Video: <u>Study Review and Treatment Applications for Shoulder Pain</u>

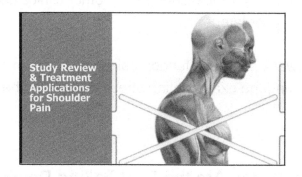

Big Questions - Who is Getting Overworked & Why?
The relevant question for locating the source of your pain should be: "Which joints and tissues did your body choose to overload?" Some positions and mechanics overload the front of the shoulder, some overload the back, while other positions overload the neck and upper back.

Forward slouching postures are the first step in creating scapular dyskinesis.

Thoracic Spine & Shoulder Pain
The upper back is anatomically known as the thoracic spine. The thoracic spine is unique because it has enlarged transverse processes for articulations for the ribs. Simply put, the spine has places for the ribs to attach and stabilize. The ribs move

when we breath, turn, and twist. They are also sites for muscle attachments.

The thoracic spinal curves are important in maintaining center of gravity. The bowling ball of a head should sit above the shoulders and hips. When the head position moves forward, it changes the thoracic and lumbar curvatures and stress forces are transferred to other areas of the body. The amount of slouch and lean determines where the forces accumulate and the tissue that has to respond.

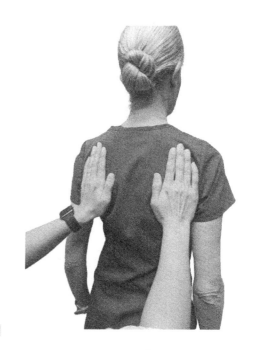

Most chronic repetitive stress injuries occur when abnormal stress is placed upon a tissue not designed to handle that stress in the specific position. Slouching will overload spinal joints, muscles, tendons, and ligaments.

Slouching changes the scapula position and glenohumeral joint position even more. A forward-leaning and rounded shoulder posture significantly alters the forces on shoulder muscles and tendons.

Forward-leaning postures place excessive strain on the shoulder tissues.

Decreased Thoracic Extension & Shoulder Pain

Thoracic spine position is one of the factors determining scapular position. Excessive forward flexion is hard on shoulders. A lack of thoracic extension also changes forces across the shoulder and limits the ability to raise the hand of the head.

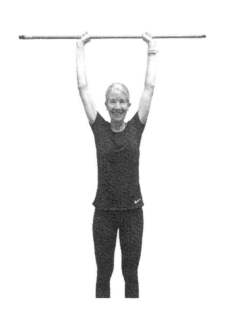

Try This

Try sitting in a chair in a neutral position; basically your best posture position if a crazy nun with a ruler was threatening you. Raise your right arm above your head. Then slouch forward and raise the hand. Next, try extending the thoracic spine backwards as much as possible and raise the hand. The relative position of the hand changes significantly with each thoracic position.

Thoracic spine function is essential to shoulder function. To prove this, next time you are in the kitchen try the following test. Reach for a plate on the middle shelf of the cupboard like you normally would. Then round the thoracic spine forward and grab the same item. Then repeat with the thoracic spine extended. What did you feel in your shoulder with each position?

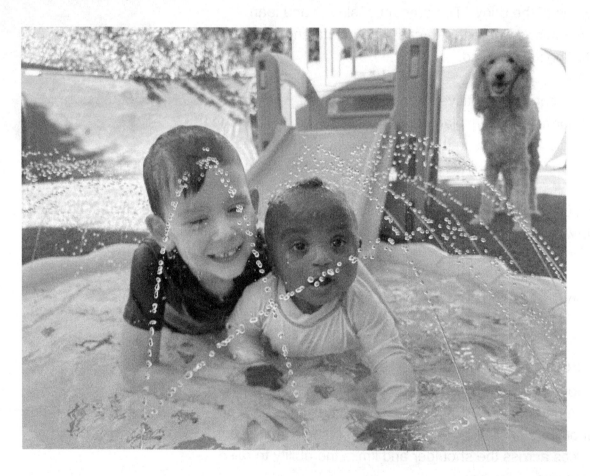

Golfers and Thoracic Spine

For fun, sit on a patio that overlooks a golf course or driving range. I realize my idea of fun is not everyone's, but try it. Especially in 50 and older communities, the golf course provides hours of entertainment. Look at the golfer's thoracic spine during their swing.

A golf swing involves a combination of pelvic and thoracic rotation with coordinated shoulder movements. A golfer's swing with excessive thoracic flexion looks very different than a golfer with a normal thoracic spine. A lack of thoracic rotation alters shoulder movements and how the swing transitions from the backswing to the follow through.

When the thoracic spine can't rotate, the golfer finds another way to swing the club. Instead of coiling in the hips and rotating the thoracic spine, they tend to sway to the side and change the clubhead's path. The altered golf swing acceleration and deceleration forces will eventually overload other tissues in the body. A lack of thoracic spine motion significantly alters a golfer's swing, power, control, and force absorption.

If you are willing to do the hard job of a prolonged happy hour on the 19th hole patio, you will see many examples of altered swing mechanics from upper cross syndrome and decreased thoracic spine mobility. They still find a way to hit the ball, but not as efficiently as possible.

The same goes for most people. They find a way to get through their activities, but not efficiently with altered thoracic spine, scapula position, and glenohumeral angle.

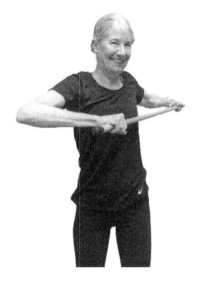

Mike Push Up Story

I once bet Mike lunch that a 13-year-old girl could do more pushups than him, and he lost!

For a little context, I once saw Mike take a 5-gallon paint bucket and shake it above his head like it was a martini. Mind you I was struggling to carry the other 5-gallon bucket from the car. He had super crazy strength. I know it is hard to believe that Mike could have been bigger and stronger then now, but he was.

A couple years later Mike was having shoulder pain that we couldn't figure out. The orthopedic and movement tests were not giving consistent results or indications. His pain was inconsistent, but we suspected something internally was damaged. The amount of shoulder muscle he had was making the diagnosis impossible.

During that time, a 13-year old girl came into the office with mom because of back pain from rowing. She was on a crew team and tweaked her back. She was smaller and had a significant power to weight ratio, not to mention her core and upper body was in great shape from rowing.

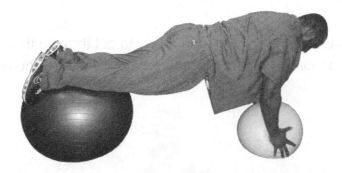

In a very crowded PT bay and in a public way, I bet Mike that she could do more pushups than him. I also increased the difficulty by having their feet be on the vibration plate shaking while the hands were on an exercise ball. Lunch at Chipotle was the bet.

Mike had to take the challenge.

We had suspected internal damage in the shoulder but we didn't have an MRI yet for confirmation. I knew he could do a bunch of pushups on the ground because we did that in the testing. So I rigged the bet by placing his feet and arms on unstable surfaces, which would require more shoulder stabilization and increased shearing forces on the labrum.

Mike fought his way through 15, and of course she did a bunch of pushups. His shoulder couldn't handle the combination of weight, instability, and shearing forces in that position.

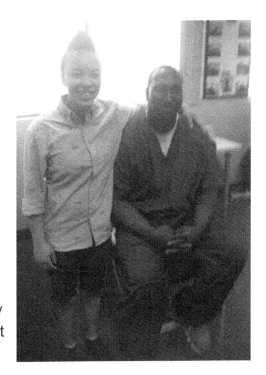

The MRI and surgery did find significant labral damage, and the surgeon was amazed how Mike was functioning with that much damage to the internal structures. His massive shoulder muscles were compensating to protect the shoulder during the day, but couldn't keep up lifting or functional exercises.

Lunch was really good, but getting to tell the story over and over about Mike losing a pushup contest to a 13-year-old has been priceless.

Video: Mike Push Up Story

Chapter 11: Scapular Dyskinesis & SICK Scapula

The Scapula

There is a beautiful subtlety to how the scapula functions with every posture and movement for the upper extremity. It also plays a vital role in the thoracic and lumbar spine posture and movements. The position of the scapula allows specific muscles to stabilize and also transfer energy during movement. Slight alterations to thoracic blade position lead to many back and neck injuries.

In addition to helping support the head through the trapezius and levator scapulae muscles, the scapula and its position is critical to supporting and moving the shoulder. Most people do not appreciate its function in transferring explosive power from the pelvis and core to the arm for a baseball pitch or tennis serve.

Minute changes to the stability and position of the scapula alters arm function and stress loads across the supporting soft tissue. Over time and repetitive injuries, these changes get worse and finally noticeable to the eye. By this time a professional baseball player would either be injured or benched because of his loss of control and stamina. His function would have been his downfall before the physical and visual changes would have been seen by the average person.

SICK Scapulae is an acronym:
Scapular malposition
Inferior medial border prominence
Coracoid pain
Kinesis abnormalities (scapular dyskinesis)

The first part of the acronym refers to the position of the scapula being lifted upward toward the ear and rounding forward. It is sitting at an incorrect position (malposition). Soft tissue injuries and tenderness increase around the borders of the scapula and muscle insertions of the rhomboids, serratus, and trapezius muscles along the inside and top of the scapula. The pectoralis minor, coracobrachialis, and short head of the biceps all attach to the coracoid process on the scapula, which is why it becomes tender.

The last part of the acronym refers to how the scapula moves, not just with one repetition but with repeated activity. The initial starting position at rest is altered or in a less than ideal position. Additionally, the muscles that support and try to stabilize the scapula during movement are unable to properly function, especially with repeated activity and muscle fatigue. The problem usually gets worse with repeated forceful activity.

Scapular dyskinesis is a problem with either the shoulder blade position and ability to anchor the shoulder during motion.

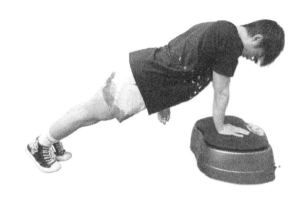

The fancy scrabble term dyskinesis means altered movement. For the shoulder joint, the altered movements are less than ideal, which changes stress loads on other tissue or makes the upper extremity movement system less effective. The changing scapula positions also changes the glenohumeral joint angle, which can lead to labral or impingement injuries

Return to the image of shooting a cannon of a canoe. As the stabilization platform shifts from a stable concrete base to an unstable canoe, the accuracy and efficiency of the cannon decreases.

As the condition worsens, people experience increasing:
- Pain along the scapula borders
- Weakness and fatigue with movements
- Decreasing range of motion, especially above the head
- Snapping or clicking of the scapula on the ribs with movement
- Scapular winging
- Forward rounded shoulders and posture changes

People most commonly describe pain and tenderness around the scapula, especially along the medial (inside) border and top. They feel fatigue from vigorous or repetitive activity. They fatigue easily when working with their hands above their heads.

Consider the muscular component for a second. We have many muscles that are involved in scapular motion. Some are:
- Too short and tight
- Stretched and less able to properly contribute to stability
- Weak
- Overactive

Neurologically, we could have nerve damage to some of the muscles, which is more common with trauma. In older adults without recent trauma, this is less likely the case. Usually we are seeing a combination of poor neuromuscular control and movement patterns.

Years of poor posture, poor movement patterns, changing spinal positions, weakening muscles, and compensating overdominance of muscles leads to scapular dyskinesis.

Scapular Dyskinesis Is a System Problem

Older adults are experiencing a series of system failures that they eventually cannot compensate for any longer, leading to shoulder and back pain. System problems need system treatments. Correct the biggest and most painful problem first, but start laying the groundwork for long term system improvement.

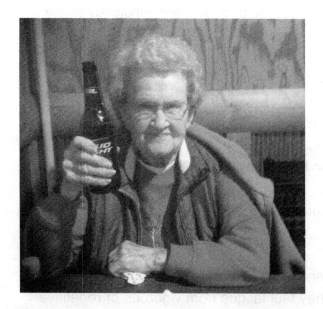

Grandma Ardy always says to enjoy a cold beer after a hard day of exercises.

Old Man's Driving and SICK Scapulae

SICK scapula syndrome (scapular dyskinesis) is a system failure or dysfunction. The system doesn't work well or do what it is supposed to for long periods of time. It can do its job for a minute or two, but not for long periods of time.

System failures are not any one problem. They are a combination of problems that all make each other that much worse. So much like my dad's driving.

I taught my four-year-old son to call my dad "Old Man" instead of grandpa, mainly because it drives my dad nuts. One day Max asked me, "Is the Old Man a bad driver because he rolls on red and drives too fast?"

I responded, "yes, and other things."

Max: "Because he talks on the phone even when you get mad at him?"

"That too. He also slows down on the interstate when he talks, gets easily distracted, and doesn't check his blind spot before he changes lanes. Blinkers are erratic. He also tailgates and texts while driving."

Max: "Has Old Man gotten more speeding tickets than you?"

Me: "Yes dude, a lot more."

Max: "Mom says you get more speeding tickets than her."

Me: "That's true. But she also uses the carefully worded phrase that she hasn't received any 'moving violations' or accidents. Mom has her stories, but she is a much better driver than Old Man."

Max: "Would Old Man be a good driver if he didn't talk on the phone or roll on red?"

Me: "No, he would still be a bad driver."

Max: "Is Old Man a bad driver because he makes lots of bad decisions?"

Me: "Yes, Max. It isn't any one bad decision but a bunch of bad decisions that makes him a bad driver."

Max: "Can we get ice cream because we are good drivers?"

Me: "Of course, dude, just don't tell Mom."

Max: "Snitches get stitches."

System failures are a combination of things. There isn't any one thing that makes the system fail. A combination of dysfunction leads to an overwhelming system failure.

Just like Old Man. A lot of things make him a bad driver. Fixing any one thing will not improve the overall system failure. The combination of multiple factors is what makes him a bad driver.

Public Safety Announcement: *Sun Lakes residents are advised to avoid a red full-sized pickup with Montana plates and a Seattle Seahawks license plate frame.*

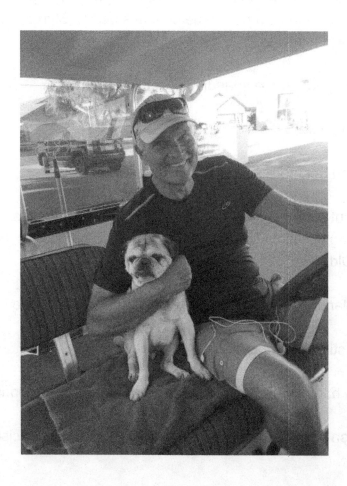

Chapter 12: Healing Process

Enhancing the Healing Process

In order to understand how and why various treatments work, it's important to be familiar with three stages of healing: inflammation, proliferation, and maturation.

The first phase, *inflammation* occurs immediately after the injury. The area becomes red and swollen, is tender to the touch, and range of motion is reduced. The purpose of inflammation is to prepare the area for healing. Many individuals believe that inflammation is abnormal following an injury and that it prevents the healing process when the opposite is actually true. The damaged tissues are sending a red alert to the body, signaling the need for cell repair and proliferation.

The second phase, called *proliferation,* is when the actual healing begins. Fibroblasts (repair cells) move to the injury area and begin to produce scar tissue. Scar tissue can form relatively quickly and protects the area from further injury. Scar tissue is type III collagen, which is meant to be a quick patch. I previously described this quick patch as "the body's duct tape." However, it lacks the elasticity and strength of type I collagen that should eventually replace it when the injury heals correctly.

During the final *maturation* phase, scar tissue in the area is replaced with healthy type I collagen. At the same time, a new blood supply is delivered to the injured area as small veins and capillaries that may have been damaged heal or are replaced. At this point, the injured area should function as it did before the injury occurred.

When something interrupts the healing process, it fails to completely repair. The injury can become chronic, along with the pain that accompanies it. This can happen for a variety of reasons including infection, decreased nutrient flow, and sometimes the body just doesn't fix the area right the first time.

Ever have those projects that get started but never completely finished? You started with the best intentions but somewhere along the process you become distracted or something else comes up instead. Then you never went back to completely finish. The same thing happens to the body with healing. It starts with a quick patch but does not

come back to break down the patch and replace it with proper tissue.
Many times improper healing is due to re-irritation of the injured area. Basically you start challenging the region before it is ready to handle it. This is especially common in muscle and tendon chronic repetitive stress injuries.

If the injury gets "stuck" in the middle of the healing process, chances are that the tissues involved will not recover correctly without some sort of intervention. Sometimes this means breaking up the scar tissue that is preventing the influx of proper healing.

Tendonosis is the proper term for this low grade tendon injury. Tendonitis involves higher levels of active inflammation which occurs with trauma and sudden injuries. Low grade chronic aggravations and injuries are more likely to be tendonosis. There is an injury but not the inflammatory cells that occur with an acute injury or injection.

Tendinopathy is pain and reduced function of tendons. Often the injury is due to the culmination of multiple injury processes rather than a single event. The chronic repetitive stress leads to loss of tissue integrity and subsequent tearing or rupture.

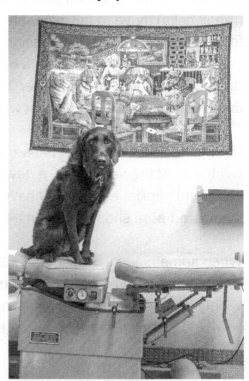

I like to compare chronic repetitive injuries as adding pennies to a penny jar. Some days you add 15 pennies, some days you take out five pennies. Over time there is a tendency to add more pennies than you are removing, and eventually the jar starts to overflow. The overflowing penny jar is your chronic repetitive stress injury. There was not a single event or day that filled the jar; instead, the jar became full after an accumulation of days and pennies.

We use different treatment strategies to make the area heal as it should have the first time.

Treatments for Specific Goals

A treatment plan for low back injuries involves utilizing specific treatments for specific outcomes. I have compared utilizing a combination of treatments to having a tool box full of tools instead of only a hammer. More tools means more options. Some tools are better suited for specific projects.

Great treatments and plans improve all of the goals:
Pain-free Range of Motion
Flexibility
Strength
Endurance
Joint Stabilization
System Stabilization

The following treatments are how we reach the above goals. Different treatments can be utilized at different times for low back injuries. A combination of treatments is always better than any single treatment.

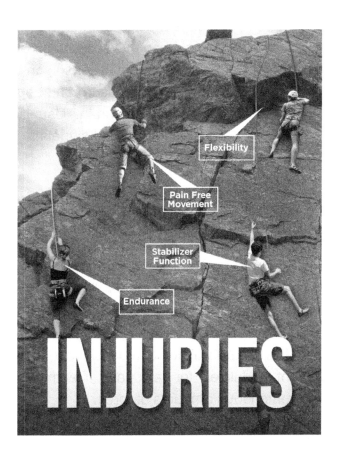

Chapter 13: Chiropractic Adjustments

My Rusty Door Hinge Theory to Describe Stuck Joint Treatments

The rusty door hinge is my personal phrase for explaining stuck and sore joints. We are all familiar with a rusty door hinge that locks up and prevents movement. We have all had a yard gate that rusts over with winter months. It takes a fair amount of work rocking the gate to restore movement to the hinge and break the rust.

To break the rust, we have several options.
1. We can very gently begin to rock the hinge, adding more and more force until it starts to move.
2. We could give several small kicks to the gate to break the rust.
3. We could give a giant kick to the gate and see if it breaks either the rust or the gate in the process.

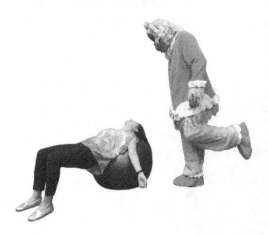

Most patients prefer not to be kicked when they are in severe amounts of pain, but the theory does correlate with joint pain and motion. When joints are injured, the muscles that guard the joints begin to spasm and prevent movement. There are small sensors in the joint that sense the increased pressure and begin to send pain signals to the brain. Usually, movement sensors in the joints send signals to the brain saying everything is okay.

This is often the cause of back pain. When joints do not move, the signal that travels to the brain says, "Ouch, I'm hurting!" The brain responds by causing back muscles to spasm to protect the joint. However, more muscle spasms cause an increased jamming of the joint surfaces and increased pain signals to the brain. This process creates a feedback loop of more spasms and pain. The cycle will continue until something breaks the feedback loop, allowing for joint movement.

Since the Arizona Chiropractic Board will not let me kick patients, we instead use several "approved treatment modalities" for back pain. Treatments allow movement in the joint without exerting tremendous amounts of force.

Watch the Video:
Types of Chiropractic Treatments For Low Back Pain

What Is a Chiropractic Adjustment?
Simply put, a chiropractic adjustment is getting a stuck joint moving. When a joint is injured, it ends up being "locked up" or "jammed together" by the protective muscle spasms. When a joint does not move, it sends pain signals to the brain.

The adjustment establishes normal joint movement and stops the pain signals. This is why people feel better after an adjustment, normal motion and decreased pain. The people who tell stories of one good crack and pain free were probably suffering from one mildly stuck joint that was sending an excessive number of pain signals. Opening up the joint relieved the intense pain. These events are less common, especially with older adults.

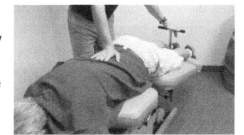

Types of Chiropractic Adjustments
These include:
- **Manual adjustments** - the traditional crack and pop method.
- **Activator Technique** - spring loaded or electric instruments that "tap" the joint.
- **Drop Table** - tables that drop, giving the provider a mechanical advantage.
- **Flexion Distraction** - utilizing a table that bends and stretches the low back.

Further descriptions and videos can be found at:
https://www.robertsonfamilychiro.com/Chiropractic-Manipulation-Different-Types-of-Chiropractic-Adjustive-Techniques.htm

The goal is to get a stuck joint moving. To the joint, it does not matter how it gets moving, just as long as motion is established. One type of adjustment technique is not better than the others. It all comes down to what works best on you.

Usually the best technique is the one that the patient feels the most comfortable with. If a patient is guarded and protective, the adjustment will not go very well.

In my office we utilize a lot of different techniques and strategies to increase joint motion. We try to do what the patient prefers, but sometimes we have to start with the gentlest approach and work toward manual adjustments.

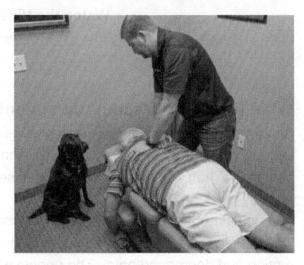

Many of our older patients started out with manual chiropractic and have always had their adjustments performed this way. With time, age, and degeneration, the body loses flexibility and its normal movements. Manual adjustments become more difficult for the patient. We transition some of these patients to less aggressive techniques such as flexion distraction, Activator Technique, or Drop Table, so they can experience the same results with less discomfort.

It is difficult to get patients to understand that successful joint movement does not depend on a popping sound. Some patients like to hear the popping sounds while others do not, but an audible pop does not determine a successful treatment.

Video:

Movement Blocks Pain

What is the Popping Sound?
When a stuck joint opens quickly it can produce an audible click or popping sound, caused by a sudden decrease in pressure within the joint. Muscle spasms across a stuck and painful joint increase the pressure inside it. This pressure causes tiny gas bubbles to be driven into the liquid inside the joint (synovial fluid). As joint space volume increases, the pressure decreases, and the gas bubbles move from the liquid and into the air space. The gas bubbles crossing the liquid-air barrier release the "popping" sound. This is the same reason a pressurized can of soda "pops" when the carbon dioxide bubbles escape back into the air after the can is opened.

Are Adjustments Dangerous? I heard…

YouTube has highlighted some of my colleagues who make poor decisions and use excessive force during adjustments, and even they have not killed anyone.

People have heard of a friend's, brother's, uncle's barber who was killed by a chiropractor. However, nobody actually knows anyone first hand. The risk of a serious injury caused by a chiropractor is somewhere between one in two million to 5.8 million, depending on the study.

I would be more likely to get seriously injured during my drive to the office today than by a chiropractor. In fact, studies have shown that the best estimates of the odds of suffering a serious complication from a chiropractic neck treatment are the same odds a person faces of dying in a commercial airline crash.

This is why my malpractice insurance is lower than most car payments.

What people should say is, "I know a lot of people who really like their chiropractor, some who have had a bad experience from a not very good one, and some people who just hate them without reason."

For more information visit:
http://www.acatoday.org/patients-why-choose-chiropractic-chiropractic-a-safe-treatment-option

No But My Friend's, Brother's, Uncle's, Barber Had a Stroke

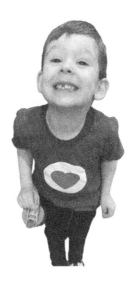

Strokes happen, and people seek treatment when they are having the worst headache of their lives. Studies have shown an increased association between vertebrobasilar artery system strokes and visits to primary care physicians. This is due to the fact that people seek treatment when they have strokes or the early symptoms of a progressing cardiovascular incident.

A (2015) study published in the *Journal of Chiropractic Manipulative Therapy* titled, "Chiropractic care and the risk of vertebrobasilar stroke: results of a case–control study in U.S.

commercial and Medicare Advantage populations" reviewed the data from 2011 to 2013.

> We found no significant association between exposure to chiropractic care and the risk of VBA (vertebrobasilar artery) stroke. We conclude that manipulation is an unlikely cause of VBA stroke. The positive association between primary care physician (PCP) visits and VBA stroke is most likely due to patient decisions to seek care for the symptoms (headache and neck pain) of arterial dissection. We further conclude that using chiropractic visits as a measure of exposure to manipulation may result in unreliable estimates of the strength of association with the occurrence of VBA stroke."
> https://www.ncbi.nlm.nih.gov/pmc/articles/PMC4470078/

The study also concluded that there was not a correlation between these strokes and visits to a chiropractic office. Would you say your primary care physician causes strokes? Of course not. Sick people seek treatment. People with headaches seek relief, and if they have been to a chiropractor before, they are likely to return for treatment thinking they just have a bad headache. It's similar to saying that people are killed at hospitals; dying people go to hospitals for help!

A bad coroner makes the news by saying a person died because of the chiropractor. However, the retraction does not make headlines when the case is properly evaluated by experts who look at the timing of symptoms, progression, or when they saw the chiropractor. I saw one supposed incident in which the coroner blamed it on a chiropractic adjustment a month before the stroke (and the patient only had his low back adjusted, not his neck). In another case, the person had a stroke in the chiropractic office waiting room, before she was ever seen. Always read the entire story.

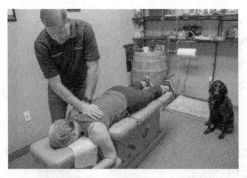

Summarizing Risks of Adjustments

The risks associated with chiropractic adjustments are extremely low, especially if the provider and patient are smart. With older patients with degenerative changes, manual manipulation may not be the best treatment. I like to say that a patient "has grown out of it." It might be a better idea to transition to the lower force and neutral spine techniques, especially drop table or Activator. If older patients have cardiovascular issues, why take the unnecessary risk of forceful adjustments?

Chiropractors & Physical Therapists

Are Chiropractors & Physical Therapists Similar?
In some ways yes, in others no. At one extreme is a traditional chiropractor who only utilizes chiropractic adjustments to treat. At the other end are physical therapists who treat using very basic exercises, stretches, and modalities.

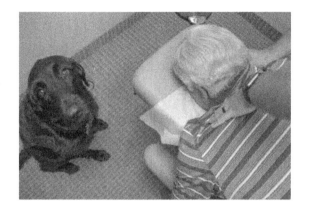

A growing group of providers blend the two skill sets. In the middle of the spectrum are chiropractors with a muscular focus incorporating soft tissue and physical therapy principles, as well as physical therapists incorporating joint movement principles. Some offices do a fantastic job of combining the best from both chiropractic and physical therapy into patient's treatment plans. Once again, the more tools in the tool box the more options for treatment.

What Does a Physical Therapist Do?
A physical therapist works to increase flexibility, strength, endurance, and joint stability through a series of exercises and stretches. Physical therapy has traditionally focused on how muscles move the body and enhance joint stability. Physical therapy involves a combination of treatments and modalities such as assisted, passive, dynamic stretching, functional exercise, fascial release, and massage.

They Are Very Different, Too!
Physical therapy is a very broad profession, ranging from inpatient stroke rehabilitation to professional sports teams, and including joint replacements, pediatrics, seniors, or general therapy clinics. Each specialty requires a different skill set.

Treatment at a professional sports clinic is very different than at a general therapy clinic. Principles are the same, but the application, progression, and outcome expectations are different.

Clinics Settings Limit & Enhance Rehabilitation

How a clinic operates, its resources, staff, and organization either limit or enhance a therapists' treatment options. Some clinic systems have standardized treatment protocols like an assembly line. They may not provide much soft tissue work or therapist one-on-one interaction. Other clinics give the therapist more leeway with office resources and time to customize treatment plans.

The reality is that some patients will do well with a standardized assembly line clinic if they have an uncomplicated injury that requires a little pain management, basic exercises, and stretches. However, if the person does not improve or experiences recurring injuries, he or she should seek more specialized treatment.

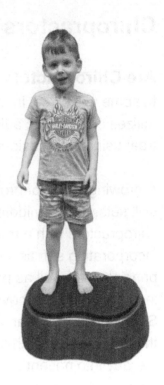

Video:

Types of Low Back Treatments

Chapter 14: Conservative Therapy

Multiple treatments can help decrease pain and inflammation. The therapeutic modalities people are most familiar with include ultrasound, heat, ice, traction, and electric therapy. These will initially control the pain.

Light motion and movement help block the pain signals traveling to the brain and enhance pain-free movement. We will give you a worksheet, diagram, or website pages of exercises.

The above treatments are the first phase, and you should progress from this point quickly. If you are in severe pain you will stay in this phase of treatment longer, but you will need to progress to the treatments that provide "the bang for your buck." If after a few weeks in a clinic you notice every other back patient is doing the exact same thing as the first week, **leave now!**

If you have severe back pain, exercises begin without weights. With improvement, we can add light resistance movement with elastic bands or rubber bands. These carry minimal risk of aggravating your back pain. We give you these exercises because you can do them at home with a simple and inexpensive rubber band to enhance strength and neuromuscular control. No expensive equipment required.

If this is where your treatment progression has stopped in the past, it's better than some offices. But it's still not great.

The next progression integrates more active therapeutic exercises. Some teach the neuromuscular and proprioceptive systems in the brain to work together again. Bridging exercises on the back and exercise ball are starter exercises. Other exercises focus on back extensor muscles. McKenzie exercises are a series of positioning exercises for lumbar disc injuries. There are standing balance exercises that make the lower extremity, hip, back, and core muscles work together.

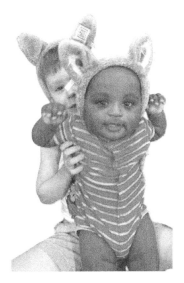

I compare this stage of treatment to building the base of a pyramid. You have to have a solid and strong foundation to build upon it. If you skip steps or fail to master each level, you will not have a strong foundation. This will catch up with you later and you will stop improving.

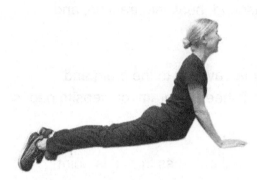

Before we get to the next level of exercises, I want to discuss more about treatments for addressing the soft tissue injuries in the back.

A July 2019 article published in the *Journal of Physical Therapy Sciences*, "Effects of McKenzie and Stabilization Exercises in Reducing Pain Intensity and Functional Disability in Individuals with Nonspecific Chronic Low Back Pain: A Systemic Review," found that McKenzie and stabilization exercises work better than conventional exercises for reducing functional disability in patients with chronic nonspecific low back pain.
https://www.ncbi.nlm.nih.gov/pmc/articles/PMC6642883/

Both Mckenzie and spinal stabilization exercises are effective at reducing low back pain and functional limitations. Each accomplish the results through increasing spinal stabilization strength and endurance, and more importantly, improving how the low back muscles work together.

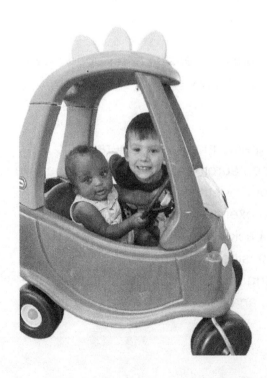

Chapter 15: Soft Tissue Treatments

Chronic Muscle and Tendon Pain Treatments

Muscles, tendons, and ligaments can become damaged over time with repetitive overuse. People like to assume these tissues heal similar to bone; that everything eventually returns to pre-injury status. Unfortunately, that is not the case. Often tissue develops scar tissue or fascial adhesions, which become weak points prone to reinjury during the next stressful event.

Besides traditional physical therapy treatments, other treatments to speed up healing include:
- Graston Technique
- Shockwave Therapy
- Class IV Cold Laser

Before learning more about these treatments, you need to understand how scar tissue functions in the body.

What Are Scar Tissue and Fascial Adhesions?

Scar tissue forms when tissue does not heal correctly, or is under chronic repetitive stress. Scar tissue is weaker than normal muscle and connective tissue; that is why it becomes chronically sore with activity.

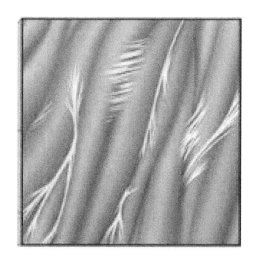

Think of scar tissue as the body's duct tape; a short term patch that supports tissue while healing. In some cases, the scar tissue is not replaced with normal type I collagen fibers. Instead, a weaker type III collagen replaces the scar tissue and "duct tape."

Fascial adhesions are another term for scar tissue. Adhesions cause restrictions between the body's fascia. Stiffness, loss of normal range of motion, and chronic pain develop from the type III collagen patches.

When a scar tissue patch undergoes stress or strain, it becomes aggravated. This process causes more scar tissue to form outside of the original patch. The process repeats itself over and over, leading to larger scar tissue patches.

I like to describe these scar tissue patches as "onions." Scar tissue grows in layers around the initial injury. Stress to the area aggravates the outside layers and causes another layer to form. The layers further from the center are easier to aggravate than the inside layers; this is why the onion continues to grow in size without the injured area healing.

Think about chronic back pain: the same weak spot always flares up in your low back. Over the years, pain always seems to start in the same place. This source of continued pain is a scar tissue onion, or weak spot that keeps flaring up.

Muscle Injury Tissue Progression

Pre-Injury	Injured	Poor Healing	Scar Tissue
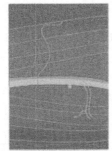	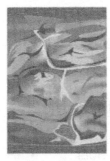	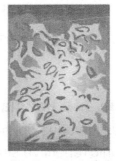	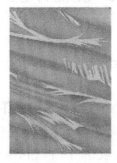
Healthy Muscle Fibers	Damaged Fibers Beginning to Heal	Scar Tissue Instead of Muscle Fibers	Muscle Fibers Limited by Scar Tissue

Causes of Scar Tissue Formation

Four common causes of scar tissue formation include:
1. **Trauma-** Sudden accident, such as stepping off a curb or falling off a ladder.
2. **Repetitive Motion Injury-** Same motion over and over.
3. **Improper Mechanics-** Slouching at a computer makes certain muscles work harder to hold up your head, neck, and shoulders.
4. **Aging-** Years of wear and tear on the body add up.

In the end, any scar tissue that limits movement and causes pain needs to be broken up to restore normal motion.

That was the simple version.

A more complex and histological description of tendinopathy would include decreased oxygen and blood flow to the injured area. Oxidative stress decreases tissue repair and increases inflammatory cytokines. Tenocytes can produce substance P, catecholamines, glutamate, and acetylcholine. These are all substances released in response to injury that increase pain and affect healing.

Some tissue cells play a role in tendon repair. Tenocytes within the tendon and sheath activate healing. Neutrophils and macrophages play a role in removing tissue debris and releasing chemicals that lead to the next phase of tissue repair.

The weaker scar tissue patch is made of type III collagen. In an ideal situation, the next repair phase transitions the type III to type I collagen, and this can continue for years beyond the original injury.

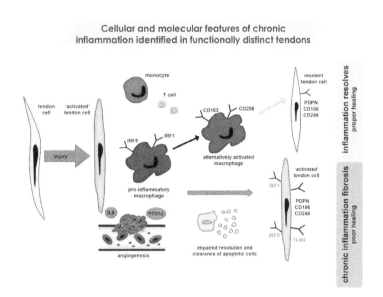

Video: Shockwave Therapy for Tendon Injuries

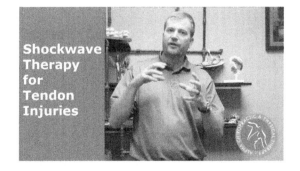

Is One Therapy Better Than Another for Chronic Tendinopathy?

No single therapy is consistently more effective than others. It all depends on the patient.

Multiple therapies such as shockwave therapy and Graston Technique are sometimes required for chronic tendinopathy to repair and heal. Proper treatment and rehabilitation of tendinopathy injuries incorporates exercises and stretches to increase muscle flexibility and strength. We retrain the body to use those muscles properly again. Muscle pattern and joint stability exercises can help prevent future injuries.

Video: Chronic Low Back Pain Reaction to Graston Technique

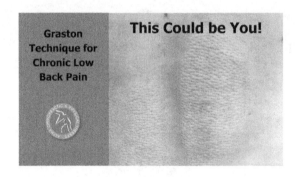

Chapter 16: Graston Technique
- Tissue Repair, Flexibility, & Pain Free Range of Motion

Graston Technique is a method of applying shear force to an injured area using specially designed stainless steel tools to break up scar tissue and promote healing.

Since its invention, Graston Technique has been shown to speed up healing of both acute and chronic injuries. In a university study, it also significantly improved range of motion in a group of uninjured college athletes when combined with a TheraBand stretching and strengthening program (Heinecke et al., 2014).

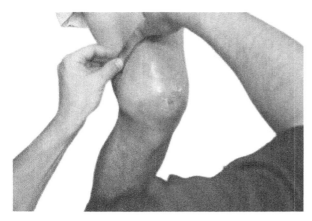

Sliding the tool on the skin creates shearing forces, which breaks up scar tissue in muscles, ligaments, tendons, or fascia. Back to the onion example, Graston Technique is using shear force to rip the top layer of the onion apart and trigger the body's repair mechanisms.

Treatment should not be overly painful. My rule is the treatment should be comfortably tolerable. If on a scale of 0-10, we say comfortably tolerable is a 3 or 4. If you are holding your breath or biting your tongue then it is too much. If a patient says 5, then we can lighten the pressure and make it more comfortable. On the rare occasion a patient says 1, then I get to dig a little harder.

As the treatment tool slides across the soft tissue fibrotic areas, the injury may feel bumpy or sandpaper-like. Redness and mild swelling may develop with treatment, especially after the first few treatments. In some cases, small petechiae or bruises may develop post-treatment. Ice therapy is commonly utilized post-treatment to limit the bruising, pain, and inflammation.

Most people notice a significant difference within a few visits.

Although it is possible to apply cross frictions using the hands, the Graston tools make the process much more efficient (and the therapist's hands a lot less sore). Thanks to their different shapes, the stainless steel tools enable the therapist to target deep tissue very effectively.

If you were to look at healthy tendon tissue under a microscope, you would notice that the tissue is dense and that the fibers all run in the same direction. In contrast, scar tissue appears irregular and loose, with the tissue fibers running in many different directions. Scar tissue is not intended to be a "permanent fix." It's the body's way of replacing damaged, weak tissue with something durable enough to protect the injury until proper healing can occur. Think of it as the body's duct tape.

Muscle Injury Tissue Progression

Pre-Injury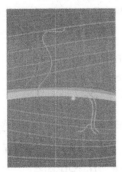
Healthy Muscle Fibers

Injured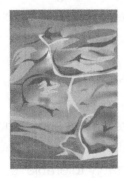
Damaged Fibers Beginning to Heal

Poor Healing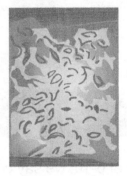
Scar Tissue Instead of Muscle Fibers

Scar Tissue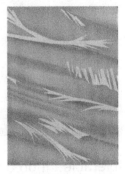
Muscle Fibers Limited by Scar Tissue

At some point, the duct tape has to come off. The therapist uses Graston to remove the temporary fix, so healthy collagen fibers can aggregate in its place. He or she does this by sliding the stainless steel tool over the injured area until it "catches" on the scar tissue, identifying the area of restriction that needs to be released.

In technical terms: Graston Technique does the following:

- Separates and breaks down collagen cross links in the scar tissue.
- Stretches the connective tissue and muscle fibers apart.
- Accelerates fibroblast activity.
- Alters maladaptive reflex patterns in the muscles that have developed in response to the chronic injury.
- Increases blood flow in and around the area.
- Increases histamine response to create swelling. This swelling signals the body to send fibroblasts and myoblasts to the area to populate it with healthy tissue.
- Increases muscle flexibility, strength, and functional movement

A word of caution here: Graston Technique is not always comfortable. Scar tissue is tough, and it takes a substantial amount of pressure to break it up. After a Graston session, you may notice swelling and bruising in the area.

I have also seen more than a few people attempt "do it yourself Graston." They do a great job of bruising the area and tearing up the skin, but not a very good job at addressing the underlying problem.

Graston Technique is a skill. I have seen a lot of providers say they do Graston Technique or any of the instrument-assisted soft treatments, and not everyone is skilled. There are only certain people I go to for soft tissue and Graston treatments because of their experience in how long, hard, deep, and when to stop. Anybody can boil water and add noodles, but not everyone is a chef.

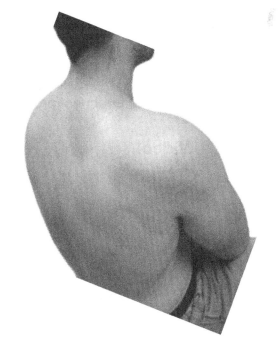

The other thing to remember about Graston is that it's proactive as opposed to reactive. It makes the healing process continue until it's properly finished. When injuries to the low back don't heal properly, the result is dysfunctional movement patterns, which, if left unaddressed, lead to bigger and more complicated injuries.

When the low back starts to lose range of motion, you will find it harder to perform activities of daily living (especially activities involving bending, twisting, or reaching), and chances are that other parts of the body will start to compensate. If left untreated, injuries that start in the low back have a way of involving the other parts of the body.

For more Information, watch the following Graston Technique Video.

Active Release Technique

Active Release Technique (A.R.T.) is a therapy similar to Graston Technique. Instead of using instruments, an A.R.T provider uses his hands to break up scar tissue. During an A.R.T. treatment, a patient will be asked to move and rotate muscles depending on the situation. The combination of movement and hand placement produces shearing forces across the muscle and fascia to break up scar tissue.

Graston Technique and A.R.T are often utilized by a provider during the same treatment. You will frequently see a provider using A.R.T concepts with the Graston Tools, mainly to reduce strain on the provider's thumbs.

Massage therapy, manual therapy, and other soft tissue treatments can also enhance treatment. Each of the soft tissue therapies has its own advantages. Every provider has his or her own preferences, and you will find a substantial difference in skill levels between soft tissue treatment providers.

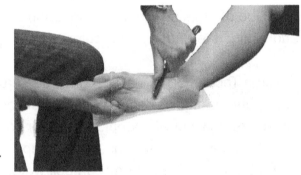

Video: Differences in Shockwave Therapy Treatments

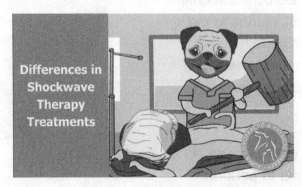

Chapter 17: Shockwave Therapy
- Tissue Repair, Flexibility, & Pain Free Range of Motion

You are probably familiar with lithotripsy: a method surgeons use to break up kidney stones. Extracorporeal shockwave therapy utilizes the same principle to break up fascial adhesions and ease muscle tightness that gets in the way of the healing process.

The shockwave instrument for musculoskeletal injuries is applied directly to the skin. The compressive energy causes tissue to stretch. Normal muscles and tendons easily stretch to the pressure, however, scar tissue does not have the elastic qualities and cannot stretch, so it ends up absorbing increasing amounts of energy and breaking the scar tissue fibers. In addition to breaking up the fascial adhesions, it improves blood flow by stimulating capillaries to regrow, bringing blood and nutrients to the tissue.

Continuing my scar tissue onion analogy. If Graston Technique is ripping the top part of the onion off and working top to bottom, shockwave is stomping on the onion and creating fractures throughout the entire onion. It helps the healing process all through the onion before Graston gets to the next layer. This is why we like to use them together when a person can handle it.

Repeated impact forces break down the scar tissue and trigger healing in the tissue. This type of treatment focuses healing in the area that needs it: the zone with excessive scar tissue that is not doing its job.

You may notice some redness or mild swelling in the injured area after a shockwave treatment. We have come to think of any inflammation as a bad thing, but remember that this is an important part of the healing process: the body's way of signaling healing cells to congregate in the area and start creating new, healthy tissue (handymen theory). We need some inflammation to trigger healing responses, but not too much which slows down the healing process.

the shockwave instrument is noisy, most patients find that shockwave is a very able treatment that yields good results in a relatively short time. The therapy is to a comfortably tolerable level.

My instructions to patients are to keep it reasonable. A comfortable biting feeling or sensation is okay but pain is not. The biting feeling is the scar tissue absorbing the energy and breaking. We are not going for pain or the most amount of discomfort a person can handle. Only bad things happen at this level, so be reasonable.

Some people have heard of calcific tendonosis, or where tendons become calcified because of excessive stress and strain. With overwhelming forces the body begins to place calcium within tendons and ligaments, most seen near the tendon to bone attachment site. Put simply, the section of the tendon contains more calcium from chronic injury and the calcium was the reaction to chronic stress and the body's attempt to strengthen the tendon.

Calcified tendons do not have the same structural elasticity as normal tendons. With some chronic injuries, calcium deposits can build up in the area and prevent normal tissue function. Calcified foot, knee, and shoulder tendons have been treated for many years with shockwave therapy to mechanically break up the calcium and trigger proper healing.

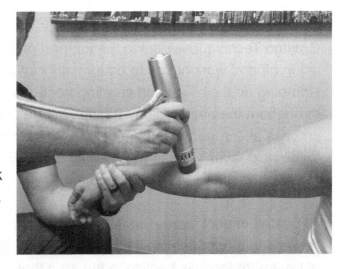

Shockwave therapy has been a fantastic addition to our office for many injuries, especially in older adults. Graston Technique can be too aggressive for some bodies and ages, but shockwave is much gentler and better handled by patients. The treatment can be gently applied and slowly increased in intensity as a person is able to handle it.

The therapy is applied to more muscles and tendons than the one that hurts. As previously discussed, the low back is a system. When a single ligament, muscle, or tendon becomes painful we utilize shockwave to enhance healing. The therapy is also applied to the other soft tissues to enhance system function and reduce future injuries.

Shockwave is especially effective for reducing muscle shortening and scar tissue in the levator scapula and upper trapezius muscles resulting from upper cross syndrome, enabling patients to help restore balance between these tightened and shortened muscles and the middle and lower back muscles that have lengthened and become weak as a result. Adding shockwave to a stretching and exercise routine can shorten rehab time and get you back to pain-free function in your daily and recreational activities.

All of the treatments can help with tendon repair. We often use Graston Technique and shockwave therapy together to treat injuries. Shockwave therapy is commonly used first on very tender or painful injuries because it is more comfortable and produces less soreness post treatment.

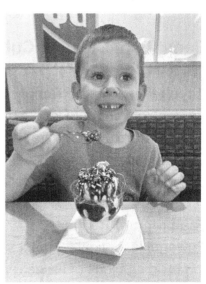

Intensity of shockwave therapy can be increased or decreased to ensure that it is always comfortable. It should not hurt. Patients are often surprised that the comfortable compression can trigger the body's healing response. Those being treated with neck and back injuries frequently feel immediate relief and improved range of motion.

Many of our older patients prefer shockwave therapy over more aggressive soft tissue treatments because it causes less bruising, especially for those on blood thinners.

The cost of the equipment and patient's cost initially made shockwave treatments unfeasible in an outpatient setting. Thankfully as technology changed, we were able to add shockwave therapy treatments at a reasonable cost.

Video: Graston Technique vs Shockwave Therapy

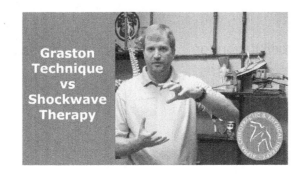

Chapter 18: Class IV Cold Laser

Significant benefits are associated with class IV cold laser. Lasers emit specific frequencies that stimulate reactions inside the cells. Different frequencies cause different actions within the tissue.

Not all lasers are equal. Different lasers have different power levels, depth of penetration, and amount of energy produced. Class IV are the newest and most powerful, and range from 10-25 Watts. Class III lasers do not offer similar benefits for severe pain and swelling. Offices with strong lasers will tell you how many Watts the laser produces per second. If they don't know, then it is probably a class III laser.

Benefits of Class IV Cold Laser

Accelerated Tissue Repair and Growth
Photons of light from lasers penetrate into tissue and accelerate cellular growth and reproduction. Laser therapy increases the energy available to cells so they can work faster, better, and quickly get rid of waste products. When cells of tendons, ligaments, and muscles are exposed to laser light, they repair and heal faster.

Faster Injury Healing
Powerful laser light increases collagen production by stimulating fibroblasts. Collagen is the building block of tissue repair and healing. Laser therapy increases fibroblast activity and therefore collagen production to speed healing.

Reduced Fibrous Tissue Formation
Low level laser therapy decreases scar tissue formation. By eliminating excessive scar tissue and encouraging proper collagen production, painful scars and chronic pain are reduced.

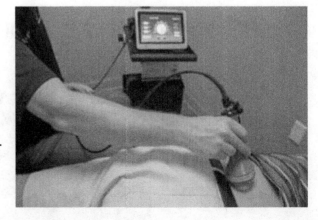

Anti-inflammation
Laser therapy causes vasodilatation, or increased blood flow. It also increases lymphatic drainage to decrease swelling or edema. Therefore laser therapy reduces swelling caused by bruising or

inflammation while speeding the recovery process.

Pain Relief
Class IV Laser therapy decreases pain by blocking pain signals to the brain. Some nerve cells sense pain and send signals to the brain. This protective mechanism can be overly stimulating, producing chronic pain and nerve sensitivity. By decreasing inflammation and edema, lasers further decrease pain sensations. Laser therapy also increases endorphins and enkephalins, which block pain signals and decrease pain sensation.

Laser therapy decreases painful nerve signals and increases mechanisms to decrease pain.

Increased Blood Flow
In the body, increased blood flow usually means faster healing. Blood carries nutrients including oxygen and ATP; and building blocks to the tissue and carries waste products away. Laser therapy increases the formation of small blood vessels or capillaries in damaged tissue.

Increased Repair and Regeneration
Laser therapy increases enzyme and metabolic activities that affect cell repair and regeneration. The enzymes are turned on "high" to speed healing.

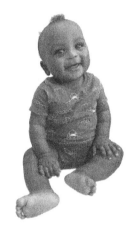

Nerve Function and Repair
Nerves can heal very slowly or have difficulty completely healing. Lasers speed up this process. Damage to specific nerves produces numbness, impaired function, or increased pain. Laser therapy treatments increase the amplitude of action potentials to restore nerve function and reduce pain.

Increased Energy Production - ATP
Certain enzymes (chromophores) can be activated to increase cellular production of ATP. ATP is "gasoline" for cells: it is the energy source that cells operate on. Injured cells often have low levels of ATP, which decreases their ability to heal and repair. By increasing ATP or "gasoline storage levels," cells have more energy to work and repair. This process is particularly important with nerve pain.

FAKTR

Functional and Kinetic Treatment in Rehab, FAKTR, is a treatment philosophy that emphasizes breaking up scar tissue and looking at the rest of the kinetic chain. Many injuries are the result of muscle, strength, or flexibility dysfunction in the kinetic chain, which leads to stress overwhelming the soft tissue. After breaking up fascial adhesions, rehabilitation and therapy provide specific exercises, stretches, proprioception, or taping to restore proper functional mechanics.

FAKTR emphasizes the kinetic chain, and treatments look for anything wrong or dysfunctional in the lower extremities or gait. FAKTR combines multiple types of treatments and thought processes for rehabilitation. It looks at solving problems in the functional system to improve your mobility.

As you have gathered by reading this book, soft tissue injuries in the back are the result of kinetic chain dysfunction. After decreasing pain and increasing tissue repair, enhancing how the system functions is the next step in the healing process.

Video: Stem Cells with Shockwave in Knee Joints - Case Study

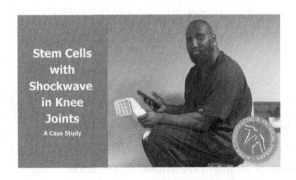

Chapter 19: Acupuncture & Dry Needling

Acupuncture

Acupuncture is an ancient Chinese medical approach to treating pain that involves triggering specific points on the skin with needles. When the needle punctures the skin, it stimulates the immune system to promote blood circulation and reduce pain.

Acupuncture Versus Dry Needling

Both acupuncture and dry needling involve inserting small, stainless steel needles into the skin. But the mechanisms behind the two therapies are different. The purpose of acupuncture is to open up a person's energy flow (also called chi or Qi), whereas dry needling is a treatment specifically designed to relieve musculoskeletal pain.

In dry needling, the therapist inserts the needles into "trigger points," which are areas of tight and injured muscle. Although these areas are often referred to as knots, they are actually micro spasms within the muscle that guard against further injury. The problem is that these knots can persist and they make the muscle shorter and less functional.

Trigger points radiate pain in distinctive patterns discussed in previous sections. Dry needling releases these trigger points to restore the muscles to their normal length and function.

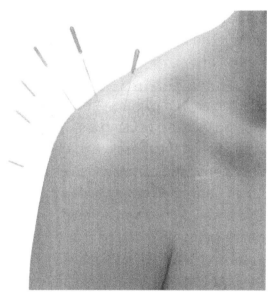

Both therapies can be effective depending on the problem. We have seen individuals with shoulder pain that we couldn't completely resolve respond to acupuncture. Acupuncture helped solve whatever was going on in their body to finally eliminate their pain and limitation.

I like dry needling for stabbing the tight muscle and getting it to relax. It will get a muscle to temporarily relax, which provides a time window for the therapist to really stretch and work an area. It helps take the muscle guarding away so the provider can provide a greater impact in rehabilitation.

Some patients have heard it breaks up scar tissue. My response is kind of, but it is not very efficient at doing so. Think of the onion, when a needle goes through an onion it will pierce the onion and create some healing. However, a therapist does not stab the onion a thousand times to really break it up. When a therapist applies a couple needles to a muscle, it is only creating a couple needles worth of damage to the scar tissue onion.

So yes, it will create a very small amount of damage to fascial adhesions and trigger some healing, but is very limited. Dry needling is much better at getting the muscles and trigger points to relax.

Or as one patient said, "it's like when my kids say they put gas in the car. They put $2.00 worth of gas into a tank that costs $70 to fill up. Yes, they put gas in the car but not enough to make a difference."

Kids these days.....

Electric Acupuncture

Electric acupuncture is a hybrid form of acupuncture that uses two needles at each insertion site to send a small electric current to the area during treatment. The feeling is similar to interferential therapy in which electrodes are applied to the skin with sticky pads. The electric current applies more stimulation to the area deeper to cause relaxation.

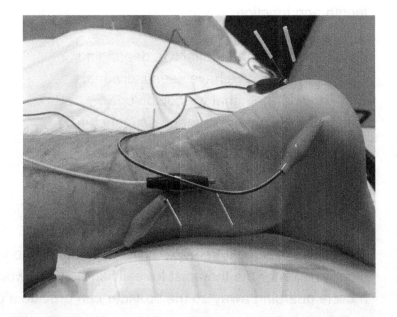

Electric acupuncture is used like electric therapy, causing a relaxation in the muscle and can get deeper into certain muscles. I had it performed on my achilles and it was a great way to help decrease some of the pain and irritation from a recent sprain. I have seen some great benefits on big, strong muscles such as the hamstring, quadriceps, and some of the glute muscles.

Chapter 20: Cupping

Cupping is a technique that utilizes cups and negative pressure to pull the tissue apart with suction. This is a therapy that began in the BC era and has continued throughout history.

Most people are familiar with dry cupping that is noninvasive. Many people first remember seeing it on Olympic swimmers and wondering what caused the red circles. There is actually a wet version that involves bloodletting and cupping. We will be discussing the dry cupping, since my state board does not allow the wet cupping.

Many people have felt musculoskeletal relief with cupping for neck, back, and knee pain. Others with headaches have seen improvement with the treatments also.

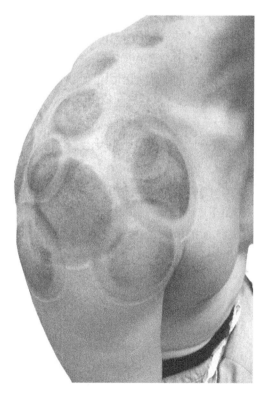

Plastic cups are placed on the skin and a suction handle removes the air, creating negative pressure and a vacuum effect. The skin can be seen pulling into the cup. With increased pressure a light or dark red can be seen with the skin inside the cup.

The negative pressure is pulling tissue apart and breaking small blood vessels in the tissue. It is proposed that the pulling tissue can break the scar tissue bonds between fascial layers and in muscles, too. Breaking tissue bonds causes a release of chemicals involved in inflammation and tissue repair. This is another treatment to trigger the body's "handymen" to move to the tissue and start repairing tissue.

I have seen patients feel significant relief from these treatments, especially along the pelvis, sacroiliac, lumbar, thoracic, scapula, and shoulder muscles.

In addition to using Graston and shockwave therapy, we also combine cupping into treatments. Cupping is another way to create tissue damage and trigger healing in back muscles and tendons.

Treatments start with placing the cups and leaving for a few minutes. If a patient responds well to cupping, then the next treatment might involve moving the cups after suctioning the air. Cocoa butter is applied to the skin to help the cups move across the back. This method adds a shearing component to the suction and breaks up more tissue underneath. Moving the cups is another treatment option for triggering the body's natural healing processes.

Cupping therapy is generally safe with very few adverse events. The red circular discoloration or bruising can be seen for a few days to a week after treatment. Most times the discoloration looks worse than it feels.

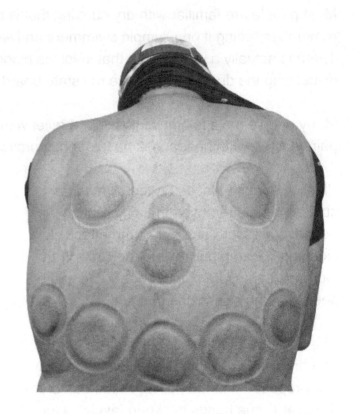

For my entertainment I once placed the cups in a smiley face pattern on my dad's back without telling him. He found out at the Sun Lakes community pool when someone started asking about the smile on his back. He was a little embarrassed and irritated with me. I reminded him that this is how kids get even with their parents, and there will be more in the future.

Video: Cupping Therapy Demonstration

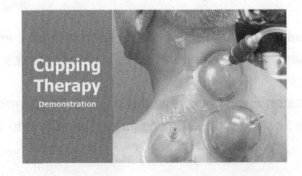

128

Chapter 21: Traction

Roller Table

Another way to help rock the join is an intersegmental traction table or roller table. The table has three large rollers that gently rock the back up and down. It is used in a pain-free range of motion, and the height is adjusted as needed.

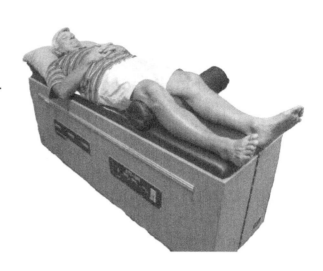

People with spinal degeneration really like this table. When you are standing, your body's weight compresses joints and jams the surfaces together. While laying on your back, the joints are in a relaxed or unloaded position. This is a very comfortable position to increase thoracic extension. The gentle rocking motions slowly move up and down the spine. After a few passes the body begins to relax the guarding muscles, allowing for more joint motion. With improvement, the roller heights can be raised to increase the spinal joint motion and extension.

Most patients really like the roller table across the upper back. It is not uncommon for a first time patient to say how much they liked it and how they didn't realize they were that stiff in their back. As the rollers continued to move up the spine they felt the relief and the improved joint motion.

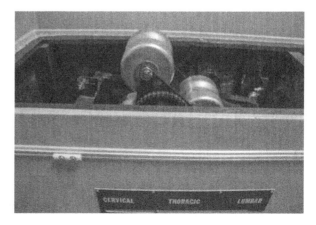

Gently rocking those joints sends normal movement signals to the brain and helps decrease our pain sensation. Treatment goals are to decrease pain and increase pain-free motion in the thoracic spine to improve shoulder mechanics. The roller table helps to "break the rust" and the muscle spasms to produce better back and shoulder movements.

Chapter 22: Spinal Decompression

Video:
Chiropractic & Disc Decompression Treatments

How Does Spinal Decompression Work?

Spinal discs have a limited blood supply requiring body movements to bring blood and nutrients to the tissue. As explained in the video above, body weight compresses joints along with the contracting lower back muscles. Nerve pain, muscle spasms, and limited movement prevent normal fluctuations in pressure that bring nutrients into the disc. Without unloading, fewer nutrients are available for disc repair and healing.

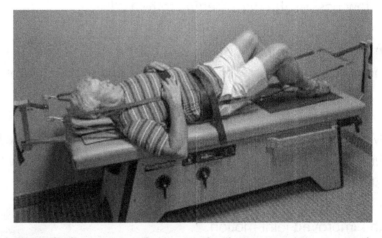

Back to the wet sponge example: With an injury, we are not moving, and therefore not creating the cycles of blood flow. It would be as if we kept a foot partially compressed on the sponge and allowed just a little bit of fluid movement.

Spinal decompression therapy pulls the foot off the sponge and lowers it down, creating a cycle that repeats over and over, enhancing nutrient flow to the disc. A specially-designed traction table pulls the joints apart, decreasing pressure on the disc. As the table returns to the starting position, the disc reloads and blood is pushed out of the disc.

A 30-minute treatment significantly increases cycling, and the amount of blood flowing through the discs. More blood and nutrients translates to faster healing and a shorter recovery time. By combining spinal decompression with chiropractic, physical therapy, exercises, stretching, Class IV laser, and massage therapy, we improve long-term outcomes.

Spinal decompression treatment alone would speed disc healing. However, without chiropractic and other therapies, muscles and joints could not protect the disc, increasing the risk of future injuries. Proper core strength and stabilization restores normal movement to the lower back and protects it during times of excess stress and strain.

Establishing normal muscle mechanics prevents future damage from occurring and reduces the likelihood of future injuries.

Which Injuries Respond to Disc Decompression?
Extruded, bulging, and degenerative discs respond well to the increased blood and nutrient flow from decompression treatments. Many people benefit during both acute episodes and to relieve chronic pain.

When Should I Get Spinal Disc Decompression?
If an MRI shows a significant disc extrusion or herniation, decompression treatments might be a good option. People with a history of degenerated discs, arthritic changes, or chronic low back pain often feel relief from the treatments when added to a rehabilitation program.

Can Disc Extrusions Heal Without Treatment?
Whenever the body has an injury it attempts to repair and heal itself. For an extruded disc, the body will try to "patch up" the disc over time. It will also try to break down the jelly material (nucleus pulposus) that has escaped out the back of the disc. It can take months to repair a disc and even longer to break down the jelly.

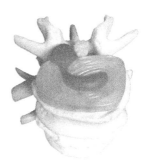

People can have disc herniations and extrusions that do not cause significant pain or symptoms, and do not require much office treatment. The risk is further tearing the fibrous disc and making the extrusion bigger before it is fully repaired.

A person could follow many of the exercises and suggestions in this book and not require treatment. However, if the disc is causing significant pain, muscle loss, or sensory changes, formal treatment is the best option.

Waiting for the disc to stop hurting and not strengthening the core muscles predisposes a person to future low back injuries. I do not recommend this option. You developed the disc damage for a reason; work on fixing the weak link in your low back and avoid this pain in the future.

Why Is Treating Disc Herniations So Difficult?

As with any injured tissue, treatment goals for a herniated disc are to decrease pain and inflammation. The location of the injury makes it difficult to treat. Every day we apply pressure to the disc—every time we take a step, twist, or sit, we stress and strain the spinal discs.

In addition, blood supply to spinal discs is very limited. In our normal movements, disc pressure fluctuates, and as a result blood rushes into and out of the area. Think of the wet sponge again: if you step on the sponge, the pressure pushes the water out of the sponge, only to rush back into the sponge when the foot is removed.

Walking provides the pressure changes needed to compress and decompress. Exercise and normal walking movements nourish a vertebral disc. When disc herniations cause severe back pain that limits your ability to walk, less blood flows to the discs. Large muscle spasms cause further compression and also restrict blood flow.

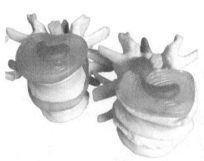

Spinal disc decompression treatments stretch the spine and decompress joints. Decompression treatment involves multiple cycles of loading and unloading the joints, as well as bringing in blood and nutrients to accelerate healing. Unloading the joints decreases pressure on the pain nerves, decreasing your discomfort.

A 2018 study published in *Spine Surgery and Related Research*, reviewed the research on chronic disc pain following surgery. In the article "Sensory Nerve Ingrowth, Cytokines, and Instability of Discogenic Low Back Pain: A Review," researchers concluded that, "Pathological mechanisms of discogenic low back pain include sensory nerve ingrowth into inner layers of the intervertebral disc, upregulation of neurotrophic factors and cytokines, and instability. Inhibition of these mechanisms is important in the treatment of discogenic low back pain."
https://www.ncbi.nlm.nih.gov/pmc/articles/PMC6698542/pdf/2432-261X-2-0011.pdf

Spinal disc pain is different from many other tissue injuries. Small tears or fissures develop in the fibrous layers of the discs. The fluid nucleus pulposus can push backwards through the tears, creating a disc bulge. Tissue damage triggers inflammatory pathways that increase disc pain nerve activity, causing increased pain nerve growth and activation in the deeper layers of the spinal disc. The herniated nucleus pulposus also activates these pain nerves.

Until the disc fibers can heal, increased numbers of pain signals travel to the spinal cord and brain. Unfortunately discs can take months to heal, especially if they experience excessive shearing forces causing more fiber damage. Even a small disc bulge can cause increased pain nerve activity for months, complicating recovery and lumbar spine function.

This is why it's essential to improve sitting, standing, and walking postures. Poor postures slow nutrient flow to the discs, delaying recovery. More importantly, slouching loads the front of the disc, causing excessive forces to push backwards on the damaged fibers. Healing can take two steps forward and then three steps back on a daily basis.

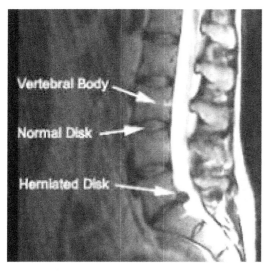

The same forces that damage spinal discs also damage the facet joints, joint capsules, spinal stabilizing spinal ligaments, muscles, and tendons near the disc. In addition, joints above and below the injury site experience increased stress as the body tries to protect the injured discs. Over time, stabilizing function in the lower back deteriorates and excessive motion damages many tissues in the lower back.

Spinal stabilization exercises target postural muscle function to minimize damaging shear forces. Extension exercises load the backs of the spinal discs, pushing the nucleus forward; away from the damaged tissues. The extension exercises help to decrease overall pain from overactive pain nerves.

A 2018 article published in the Journal of Physical Therapy Sciences, "Effects of Stabilization Exercise Using Flexi-bar on Functional Disability and Transverse Abdominis Thickness in Patients With Chronic Low Back Pain," evaluated the benefits of adding a Flexbar to core stabilization exercises. People performed 30 minutes of

exercise three times per week for six weeks.
https://www.ncbi.nlm.nih.gov/pmc/articles/PMC5857446/

One group performed stability exercises by adding a Flexbar to further challenge proprioception and stabilization. While the control group performed the same exercises without the Flexbar. Adding the Flexbar increased stimulus to the deep spinal stabilizer muscles, producing greater improvement in functional stability and reduced pain levels.

Flexbar provides a similar stimulus to the upper extremity that standing on a vibration plate does for the lower extremity.

Many people think they need to lift heavy weights to exhaustion to gain strength and endurance, but that is not true. Functional workouts often provide greater benefit to people because they challenge the weakest muscle groups and neuromuscular control systems.

Video: Whole-body Vibration Exercise and Core Stabilization in Chronic Non-Specific Low Back Pain

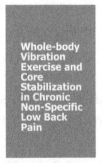 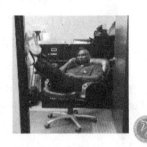 

Why Did Past Decompression Treatments Fail?

Usually when people say decompression treatments did not work for them, it is one of two reasons:

1. They flared up their sciatic pain in the first few treatments when decompression pulling was increased too fast. The back muscles did not like the stretch and spasmed to protect the back, inadvertently causing increased pressure on the disc and nerve root.

2. They went through a series of treatments that only involved decompression and the physical therapy accompanying it was lacking quality core strengthening and stability exercises. For example, a patient might say that he would go in for decompression, followed by three sets of 10 on the back extension machine, followed by a massage. The treatment was expensive and the pain returned in a few years because the person failed to stabilize his core and low back.

Spinal decompression must include proper rehabilitation exercises.

Video: <u>The Effects of Whole Body Vibration Exercise Combined with a Weight Vest in Older Adults</u>

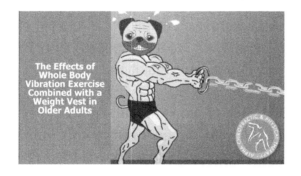

Acupuncture Instead of Disc Surgery

A 2014 article *Orthopedic Surgery* called "Traditional Chinese Medicine Treatments for Ruptured Lumbar Disc Herniation: Clinical Observations in 102 cases," showed how traditional Chinese medicine managed patient's pain without surgery. Eighty three percent of patients demonstrated partial or complete relief after two years when treated with traditional Chinese medicine. https://www.ncbi.nlm.nih.gov/pubmed/25179358

Patients showed improvement even when the disc reabsorption was not significant. To me this falls in the "just because we do not understand it doesn't mean it doesn't work" category. Eighty three percent is a really high number; this does not happen by accident. The treatments had a significant impact on those individuals, even though Western medicine does not understand the mechanisms.

Acupuncture can relieve back pain by stimulating the release of endorphins and serotonin, which changes the way the brain processes pain. It improves muscle stiffness and joint mobility by improving circulation.

Many patients utilize acupuncture to manage chronic back, neck, knee, ankle, or foot arthritis pain. Acupuncture can help reduce swelling and promotes blood flow around the lower back. We have also seen patients respond very well to acupuncture if they have chronic knee pain.

Tai Chi & Low Back Pain

A 2019 study published in *Medicina* titled "The Effects of Tai Chi Chuan Versus Core Stability Training on Lower-Limb Neuromuscular Function in Aging Individuals with Non-Specific Chronic Lower Back Pain" compared Tai Chi and core muscle work changes in the lower extremity and lower back. Both Tai Chi and core exercises improved ankle and knee range of motion and strength compared to control groups.

Improving ankle and knee strength has been shown to improve lower back pain in patients by enhancing gait and reducing spinal stress on the lower back. Each of these treatments resulted in improvement in functional activities that helped people move more easily and experience less pain. This study proved that Tai Chi is an excellent exercise for those with low back pain to improve their functional abilities for daily living activities.

Custom Orthotics

Orthotics are always difficult. Some people love theirs and others feel worse when wearing them. Custom orthotics can be very expensive, and may or may not fix the problem.

An orthotic helps to maintain and support the longitudinal arch when standing or walking. By keeping a proper arch, the orthotic prevents excessive tibial torsion and strain on the knee. It also helps to keep the femur straight, reducing strain on the hip and back. Some people will notice a significant improvement in their leg, knee, and back soreness when they wear orthotics for back pain.

Loss of foot muscle strength contributes to developing back pain. When the foot muscles are not strong enough to absorb the ground forces from walking and hold the arch in proper position, it leads to internal rotation of the knee and femur, causing excessive soft tissue strain.

Orthotics help support the foot arches by bracing the foot in proper position and limiting over pronation. However, one of the concerns with orthotic support is that the foot muscles are weakened from lack of use.

Some people really do get a great benefit by wearing orthotics. Generally speaking if the leg shows too much internal rotation and foot overpronation orthotics are worth a try. Start with the less expensive ones to see if they help, and then look for a high quality orthotic if you feel a difference.

Side Note: A good orthotic can't make up for an old and worn out shoe. I don't care how "comfortable they are."

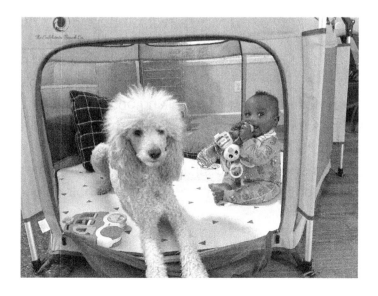

Chapter 23: Injection Therapies

Video:
Combining Pain Management and Conservative Therapy

Cortisone Injections

Cortisone injections will decrease pain and inflammation for tendon, ligament, and fascial injuries. They will block pain and inflammatory pathways and are usually effective for four to six weeks, but some people feel relief longer.

Cortisone slows down tissue repair and regeneration, which is one of the reasons a person can only have so many cortisone injections in a year. Multiple injections may increase the risk of tendon or ligament rupture. For this reason, we prefer to try other conservative treatments before introducing cortisone for mild to moderate cases.

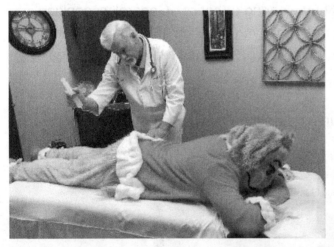

We do recommend cortisone injections for our patients when they are in severe pain, and conservative treatment is limited because of high pain levels. The injections will decrease the pain and inflammation, providing conservative treatment a window of time to enhance healing.

We also recommend cortisone injections when people are unable to be treated because of travel plans and will be walking on their feet for prolonged periods of time. The injection allows a person to enjoy his or her vacation without pain.

Other times we may recommend cortisone injections earlier in treatment include when people are unable to consistently make treatments or are unable to perform their work/home duties.

Platelet-rich Plasma (PRP)

Platelet-rich plasma is a treatment option that relieves pain by stimulating the repair machinery of the body. The platelet-rich plasma works on a very simple principle: when the platelet concentration is increased in a certain area of the body, it accelerates the healing process. Platelets contain many chemicals including:

- Glycogen
- Lysosomes
- Alpha granules
- Beta granules

To make platelet-rich plasma, a provider draws 20-30 mL of blood. The blood is then spun in a centrifuge machine for 15 minutes at 3,200 rpm. This step separates platelet-rich plasma from platelet-poor plasma. 20 mL of blood produces only 3 mL of platelet-rich plasma.

Alpha granules contain growth factors that are the main focus of platelet-rich plasma therapy. There are three stages of healing after platelet-rich plasma injection, and different types of growth factors are involved in driving different stages.

1. Inflammation phase: Lasts 2-3 days. In this phase, growth factors are released.
2. Proliferation phase: Lasts 2-4 weeks. It is vital for musculoskeletal regeneration.
3. Remodelling phase: Lasts over a year. In this phase, collagen matures and strengthens and the injury heals.

As the platelet-rich plasma technique uses the patient's own blood, the chances of an immunogenic reaction or the transfer of blood borne diseases are eliminated. Patients do experience some soreness after receiving a PRP injection.

Evidence for the use of PRP in back pain shows encouraging, safe results. However, the number of available studies is limited, especially those comparing PRP to other treatments.

Nerve Blocks

Steroid injections near the nerve root block pain and decrease inflammation where the nerve exits the spinal cord. These injections decrease pain and inflammation for several weeks to two months. Pain relief is immediate for most people, but some people will not receive any relief.

Nerve blocks are performed with special equipment in a pain management facility. Pain management physicians use MRI results and exam findings to determine the best course of treatment.

Epidural Injections

Steroid injections take place near the spinal cord, above the dura. Larger doses of medications are given to effect a larger area, as compared to a nerve block.

A great pain management facility provides tremendous relief and benefits to patients. Low back injections can reduce pain significantly. These procedures are very safe and have minimal complications.

After a patient receives an injection, his or her functional ability improves, along with our ability to enhance office treatments and exercises.

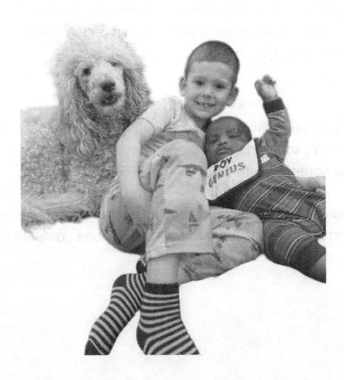

Hyaluronic Acid Injections

Video: Hyaluronic Acid & Shockwave For Knee Pain

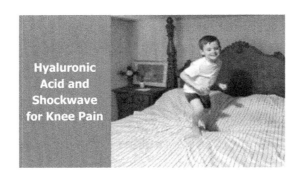

Bad backs and knees often occur together. I get asked about these injections a lot so I included this section for those who are curious. Hyaluronic acid injections, shockwave therapy, and NSIDs are common treatments for knee pain. This study looks at the effectiveness of these treatments.

In a sense the NSAIDs are for pain relief. Hyaluronic acid injections are providing a cushion to decrease pain and wear-and-tear on the knee joint structures. Shockwave therapy is ramping up repair cells for the knee muscles, tendons, ligaments, cartilage, and bone.

I've seen all three treatments provide short term relief. For medium and long term shockwave and hyaluronic injections are effective strategies for managing knee pain and promoting healing.

For long term relief, a person needs to get the painful soft tissue repaired and improve the muscle stability around the knee. Commonly that involves working the stabilizers above and below the knee in a treatment plan with home exercises.

Using these treatments can help you have less knee pain in the short term, meanwhile improving functional stability in the long term involves shockwave therapy and other soft tissue treatments.

Chapter 24: Medical Management & Treatments

- By Dr. Don Selevey NMD

Botanical-based Treatment Options for Low Back Pain:
- For **Relief of Muscle Spasms:**
  - Calcium
  - Magnesium
  - MSM (methylsulfonylmethane)
  - Homeopathic Magnesia Phosphorica
- For **Relief of Inflammation:**
  - Bromelain
  - Fish oils
  - Curcumin
  - Vitamin C
- For **Relief of Pain:**
  - White willow
  - Glucosamine sulfate (for osteoarthritis)
  - Cayenne cream
  - Medical grade DMSO (dimethyl sulfoxide; **Important:** Industrial grade is poison!)
  - Hypericum oil (St. John's Wort) – for nerve pain
  - Arnica oil – for muscle pain and spasm
  - Vitamins B_1, B_6, B_{12} and B-complex – for pain

Pharmacologic Treatment Options for Low Back Pain

OTCs: If the pain warrants some form of relief, please try to use an over-the-counter (OTC) medication. It is important to consider possible drug-drug interactions, even for use of OTCs. For example, a person with an active stomach, intestinal ulcer, renal deficiency, or pregnancy should not use an OTC that is classed as an NSAID (non-steroidal anti-inflammatory drug), such as aspirin, ibuprofen or naproxen. Acetaminophen is a different class of drug and is preferred when an NSAID is to be avoided.

Prescription Drugs

It is probably obvious that no one medication is effective in every person with low back pain (LBP). This is because there are different causes of LBP (muscle, nerve, structural) and everyone responds to medicine slightly differently, based in part on genetic make-up and in part on our past history of using medication for pain relief.

Narcotic Drugs used in treatment of LBP are usually a last resort, medically. Frankly, while drugs such as OxyContin, Vicodin, Percocet and Norco may be effective in relieving pain, the risk of side effects of the drugs often outweigh the potential benefit.

There are a couple of serious risks to consider. First, there is a risk of addiction which may lead to **a)** need for medically-supervised withdrawal, and **b)** risk of later addiction to certain street drugs, such as heroin. The "Gold Standard" for narcotic pain relief is morphine (in several forms). About 25% of patients become addicted within a few days. Heroin was once used to help reduce the amount of morphine they used – but it is just as addictive.

Later, Methadone was created to help people off of heroin; now it too is being used as a pain reliever in some people. Use of narcotics for pain relief is a vicious cycle that is best avoided.

Second, there can be an *increase* in pain with long-term narcotic use. It isn't that the body has merely become tolerant of the drug (which does happen), but that the brain's perception of pain is increased.

If you feel like you need a narcotic pain reliever, please visit a legitimate pain management center. These are often operated by Board-certified anesthesiologists who are in the best position to advise and treat with these dangerous drugs.

Our office will not initiate any form of narcotic treatment for pain management.

Non-narcotic, Prescription Drug treatment of low back pain is chosen based on a patient's history and confounding factors. For example, some prescription pain relievers are contraindicated in people with specific conditions – such as Ketorolac in women who are in later stages of pregnancy or are nursing. Commonly, a person with low back pain needs a muscle relaxant as well as an analgesic (pain reliever).

Our preferred treatment regimen for acute LBP in patients without contraindicating conditions is a combination of homeopathic *Traumeel* and *Spascupreel* and concurrent *Ketorolac tromethamine*. These are injected (two injections) into the upper, outer quadrant of the buttock. Traumeel and Ketorolac help manage pain, while Spascupreel is an anti-spasmodic agent.

Oral medications usually helpful for LBP include Diclofenac sodium and Tizanidine, for pain and muscle spasms, respectively. **Naltrexone** by mouth can be used long term for chronic pain.

Medical Marijuana

Arizona is one of the 33 states (plus the District of Columbia) that allows people to obtain and use marijuana for medical use. There are currently about 200,000 people in Arizona who are "certified" for medical marijuana use, based on a limited number of "qualifying conditions." Over 80% of these people have "severe and chronic pain" as their qualifying condition.

There are several forms of marijuana used for pain, including tropical agents, edibles, tinctures and even suppositories – in addition to smoking. Marijuana has several ingredients that have medicinal properties, although the Drug Enforcement Agency would certainly dispute this (the DEA and marijuana have a rich – and sordid – history, which colors the issue of medical marijuana).

THC is the agent responsible for psychogenic effects (the buzz or high); CBD is the agent usually attributed to pain relief. Some people claim CBD to be "better than Vicodin" but without the side-effects. Other patients say a very small amount of THC added to the CBD enhances the pain relief effect.

Medical Marijuana is always produced in a licensed facility and can be cultivated in such a way as to adjust the levels of CBD and THC to meet specifications.

For additional information about the certification process in Arizona, visit www.coppervalleymedical.com.

Hemp-based CBD

CBD derived from the hemp plant does not contain any THC, and is therefore not regarded by the DEA or local law enforcement as a controlled substance. It is available from both reputable and non-reputable sources (usually an overseas scammer), so Caveat Emptor: Let the buyer beware.

Our office usually has a small supply of hemp-based CBD from lab certified facilities available.

Chapter 25: Home Products

Different products help different people. Too many times I have said it depends on the person, and this is one of those times.

Goals of home treatments are to:
1. Decrease pain and inflammation
2. Increase flexibility
3. Increase strength

Are Inversion Tables Good?

Inversion tables are an excellent treatment tool to utilize at home as long as they are used safely and smartly. A person can apply the axial stretch to his/her arthritic joints and relieve compression forces on the disc and joints at home.

Inversion tables should not be used if a person has a difficult time reclining or hanging upside down. People with risk of stroke or significant cardiovascular disease should not use them. Check with your cardiologist or primary care physician when in doubt.

How to Use an Inversion Table

The key is to start slowly and progress steadily. Too many people try to go all the way upside-down and hang for five minutes, which is a great way to aggravate the back.

I suggest starting with a slight decline, just a little below parallel to the floor. Hang for 20-30 seconds, and then return to the starting position for 30 seconds. Repeat this process several times. Slowly begin reclining further and further over time, and slowly increasing the time to one minute.

When a person is having a bad day and feeling extra tight, it is recommended that he or she reduce the time and degree of recline. Challenging the body with too much of a stretch can set off a protective muscle spasm and "jam the sore joints together." This is how and why people flare up their backs with home inversion tables.

Is an Inversion Table Helpful for Arthritis Pain?
Some people do very well managing their daily spinal joint pain with a light inversion stretch, which takes pressure off the damaged joint surfaces. Every individual is different, and inversion is an effective home treatment for many.

Is It Good for Disc Injuries?
Most people with disc extrusions and herniations do very well with inversion tables. By stretching the joints apart, inversion relieves pressure from the compressed nerve roots. It can be a great home treatment, but be careful not to over stretch or challenge the back on a bad day.

Are Inversion Tables Good For SI & Ligament Pain?
No. Inversion tables stretch and shear the sacroiliac joint, which often makes it worse. If lumbosacral ligaments are sprained then the pulling action of inversion makes the condition worse.

Back Pain Reduces Sleep Quality
The *Korean Journal of Pain* examined sleep disturbance, depression, and pain related disability in "The Effects of Stabilization Exercises on Pain Related Disability, Sleep Disturbance, and Psychological Status of Patients with Non Specific Chronic Low Back Pain (2018)." https://www.ncbi.nlm.nih.gov/pmc/articles/PMC6037811/ Spinal stabilization exercises improved back pain and therefore also improved sleep quality. As pain decreased, the psychological conditions improved, confirmed by other studies.

Chronic low back pain has many effects on the body and quality of life. People say they can tolerate the pain, but they fail to acknowledge how the pain limits their daily activities and social behaviors. Their mood and sleep deteriorates, which has negative consequences on their personal relationships.

Do I Need to Get Rid of My Bed?
Only if it makes your pain worse. Try the guest bed or another one in the house. If you feel better when traveling or staying in a different hotel bed, then yours is probably aggravating your back.

A mattress does not last forever, and most times people try to use theirs too long. Likewise, sometimes a mattress just does not work for an individual anymore. The mattress needs to match your flexibility, weight distribution, and position at night. A bed might have been perfect three years ago, but both you and the bed have changed since then.

What Is the Best Bed?

The one that works for you. It should feel comfortable and your weight should comfortably sink into the bed. The flexibility of your cervical, thoracic, and lumbar spine determine the right bed for you. If it is too hard or soft, then excessive strain is placed on the joints.

Think of a six-year old. He or she can lay on the hard ground and their joints have the flexibility to comfortably rest without strain. As we age and lose most of that flexibility, sleeping on the ground strains the joints.

Too many times couples settle on a bed. It is not perfect for either one. When the bed softens it becomes okay for a couple years. Eventually it does not work for either person, but they do not want to replace a bed that is less than five years old.

In theory, the sleep number beds should be great. The level of firmness can be adjusted to match a person's needs. However, not every person likes them. The best bed is one that matches the individual. It is a big purchase, so do not settle.

Bed In a Box?

A bed delivered in a box to the house - how did someone come up with this idea? It works pretty well if the bed matches your flexibility. These beds also have incredible guarantees, so if you do not like it, donate the bed to charity and get your money back.

The cost is lower than many other mattresses. I have a patient who purchases one of these box beds every three years. He has chronic low back pain and this system works really well for him because just as the current bed is wearing out, another is coming in the mail. When he figured the cost over fifteen years, it is also less expensive than purchasing a more expensive bed twice.

Best Computer Chair for Back Pain?
I can slouch in a really expensive chair. The best chair is one that helps maintain your posture. The arms should be comfortably rested. The spine should be in a comfortable position to absorb forces and not place excessive strain on any joints.

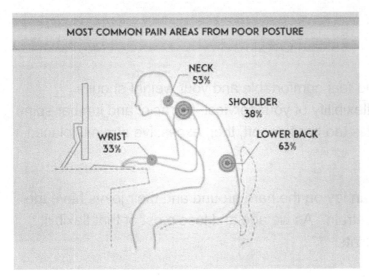

An ideal posture keeps the head above the pelvis, a line could be drawn from the ear hole straight down through the tip of the shoulder, and down to the femur's greater trochanter.

Any chair that helps to maintain proper posture is a great chair for you. A chair that encourages you to slouch is not the chair for you.

Stand Up Desk?
It took a little while, but I learned to really like standing and working. The ability to stand and change positions is helpful. I can place my foot on a small step under the desk, and further modify my back position.

A simple converter sits upon the current desk, and lifts the computer monitors to a standing position. Varidesk is the most popular name brand.

A standing workstation can be created in a book shelf, on a countertop, or on filing cabinets. Be creative in finding a solution. Keys to quality work stations are proper keyboards and computer monitor height.

Massage
Massage therapy can be a great tool for decreasing pain and muscle spasms. A good massage therapist can help relieve chronic muscle spasms and tightness, improving pain levels and flexibility. A great massage therapist can enhance your treatment and recovery.

How About Swimming?

Swimming is a great exercise for the core and lower back, especially for efficient swimmers. Muscle contraction occurs with the body floating in water. The water's buoyancy creates a non weight bearing activity with safe resistance.

Be sure that swimming doesn't aggravate the injury.

Pool running and treading water are also great activities. The best policy is to find what you like and can comfortably perform.

Video: Ice After Acute and Chronic Injuries

Ice Packs

You need a good ice pack because you should use it multiple times a day. A small three or five-inch ice pack is not going to cut it. A large ice pack can transfer a therapeutic dose of cold from the pack to the back. Also, leaning into the pack tends to push the blue gel away, so a larger ice pack can fold to increase the blue gel density. I prefer a 10-inch x 15-inch ice pack.

I tell people that icing three times a day is good, five times a day is better, and 10 times is fantastic. People are surprised but when they ice 10 times a day for a week, their back pain is significantly reduced.

Nothing decreases pain and inflammation like applying ice directly on an injury. Frozen vegetables don't cut it; they squish to the edge of the pack and do not provide direct compression to lower tissue temperature.

Do not use the solid blue ice meant to keep a cooler cold. Using those is a great way to develop frostbite through excessive tissue cooling.

Also avoid laying on your back with the ice packed between you and the bed. Many people end up falling asleep, then awake in pain and with a case of frostbite. You have been warned!

Video: Ice What Hurts

Ice Baths

Place ice in the tub, then submerge your lower back for 10-15 minutes. An ice bath decreases pain and inflammation in all of the lower back muscles and tendons. Also a great way for people in Arizona to use their pools in January.

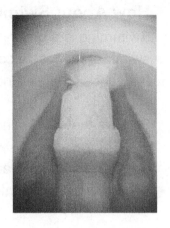

However, the worst feeling is getting stuck in the tub and unable to get out without help. This is why I do not recommend ice baths for severe lower back pain. Ice baths can be helpful for mild to moderate muscle soreness after activity.

Hot Tubs & Baths

Hot tubs can be great for providing deep heat and decreasing muscle spasms. However, heat applied after an acute injury or during an exacerbation will make it worse. Anyone who has tried this will tell you they put heat on their back at night, and then woke up in severe pain and could not get out of bed.

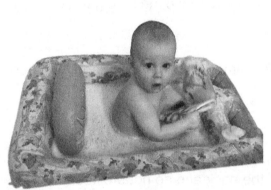

Think of a sprained ankle. Everyone knows applying ice right afterwards will decrease the swelling over the next few days. If a person put his acutely sprained ankle in a hot tub, it would accelerate the inflammatory response and swelling. The ankle would be "huge" the next day.

After the acute injury stage, hot tubs and baths are a great way to heat the lower back, hips, and leg muscles. Stretch out comfortably in the warm water and perform light range of motion exercises. If in doubt, ice afterwards to limit the potential for inflammation.

Topical Creams
Topical gels, like Biofreeze, sombra and penetrex, and some essential oils, relieve some pain, inflammation, and muscle soreness. These do not replace ice. Ice is still better. These can help relieve your symptoms and make the day more manageable. Some people like to alternate between different topicals, however it really is just personal preference. Many different products can reduce symptoms during the day and night. Oftentimes people try a variety of products until they find the ones that work for them.

Stick-on Patches
These products can be applied directly to the lower back to provide relief throughout the day. Patches can contain lidocaine or other pain relieving treatments, but they do not reduce inflammation. The warming and cooling effects can be helpful to temporarily reduce symptoms; however, the patches do not replace ice or heat packs.

Use the creams and patches to help manage daily symptoms, but remember that they are a small part of therapy. These products do not change the temperature of the skin or deeper tissue, even if they feel hot or cold. Once again, applying the pain relieving patches are not a replacement for heating or icing at home.

TENS Units
TENS units are simple home treatment devices to reduce pain. In the office, we will utilize stronger electrical devices for decreasing inflammation and blocking pain. But TENS units allow you to continue the therapy at home. The unit operates on a 9-volt battery to create an electric current that prevents pain sensors from sending pain signals to the brain.

TENS units can be used throughout the day. Many people find themselves using them both before and after activity. I prefer to use the TENS in combination with ice whenever possible. The combination blocks pain and reduces inflammation.

Home Back Massage Chairs
Home units are tricky to use during a flare up. The compression and rolling of the massage chairs can help relieve painful muscle spasms. However if you overdo it at home with the intensity or treatment time, it can lead to an exacerbation or flare up. When these chairs are used correctly and cautiously they can be a tremendous benefit and relieve daily symptoms.

Deep Tissue Massagers

Hand Held Trigger Point - These work on tight muscles and knots. Once again, *be reasonable with your force.* A little bit of compression goes a long way, too much can make it worse.

Machine Operated - Theragun is one of many brands of electric operated muscle stimulators that cause compression or vibration. These tools work on the muscles to increase recovery and relaxation. Vibration therapy decreases muscle spasms by modifying stretch receptors in tendons and muscles. Compression therapy also decreases muscle spasms in larger muscle groups. Be careful when working on smaller muscles and tendons, especially those close to the bone.

Tennis Balls - Place a tennis ball behind the lower back muscles and gluteal muscles for a light trigger point massage. Apply light compression for 10 seconds and then move to a different spot. Many people apply too much pressure, creating muscle spasms and aggravating their low back pain. Be careful and smart.

Kinesio Tape / RockTape

People are very skeptical about the stretchy tape. But the tape recruits sensory nerves to send signals to the brain regarding body postures. As we have discussed, much of treatment is trying to train the sensory system to work with the muscular system.

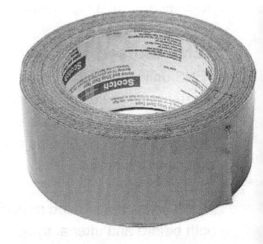

There are several kinds of neuromuscular tapes for purchase, such as kinesio tape or RockTape. Find what works for you. There are numerous YouTube videos showing how to tape for various injuries.

Taping with kinesio tape is a very effective way to reduce pain and promote healing. The tape does two things:
1. Pulls the skin around the injury up slightly to improve blood circulation in the area.
2. Triggers proprioceptors in the skin, making you more aware of movement to enhance muscular activity.

Foam Rollers

Foam rollers, available at many running specialty shops, are a great way to relieve fascial tightness and muscle tension. They require a certain amount of practice and agility to use, but they are simple, effective, and inexpensive. I like the really wide rollers (mine is about 4 feet in length), because they have a larger surface area to roll over, which is especially important for the back and shoulders.

Tennis balls, dog squeaky balls, or compression balls can be used similar to foam rollers. Place the balls against the wall and lean into them. By standing you can control the amount of pressure against the ball. Often laying on the ball can be too much pressure and aggravate the condition.

Back Braces

A simple and inexpensive brace will significantly decrease daily back pain by supporting the spine and reducing joint stress. The brace supports body weight and decreases mechanical forces through lower back discs and joints. Braces also help remind people to be careful with their movements and positions.

For people who have chronic pain, I recommend getting two braces; one to sweat in and one to wear during the day. If you wear the brace for yard work, you won't wear it during the day for normal activities. Braces can be cheap and very effective, such as the Muller Back brace for around $17 on Amazon.

Expensive Braces And Supports
There is a time and place for everything, but I do not recommend buying an expensive brace right away. Try the less expensive braces for a week or two first. In certain cases with severe injuries and disc herniations, an expensive LSO back brace is worth the cost. For the right person, it provides a tremendous benefit. For a person who only needs an inexpensive brace for a week, the money could have been better spent elsewhere.

Body Pillows
Sleeping with a pillow between the knees improves sacroiliac and hip joint angle, reducing strain on the low back. People with severe back injuries often benefit from a body pillow to lean on at night, which enables a person to modify his or her sleeping positions. Laying at an angle is one more position to rest in at night, giving a person more options for comfortable sleeping positions

Recliners
Grandpa Bud loved his Lazy-Boy Recliner: white shirt, loosened suspenders, and navy blue pants with a button undone completed his nightly ritual. It could have been that the extra lumbar support and angle decreased body weight stress through the lumbar discs and relieved lower back strain, enabling him to drift asleep. It could have also been that the long work day and very tall nightcap provided the perfect recipe for sleeping. Either way, many people feel significant relief when resting or sleeping in a recliner.

The angle of the recliner offers a different position and mechanical stress load on the lumbar spine than laying flat on the back. Many people will start sleeping in the bed, switch to the recliner after a few hours, and then go back to bed after a few hours. Find what works for you.

Exercise Balls
Every person with chronic low back pain or disc injuries needs at least one exercise ball at home. The ball can be used to decrease back pain by laying across it on your stomach or back, depending on the type of tissue injured. More importantly, the number of high quality exercises that can be performed on a $25-ball is amazing. I recommend

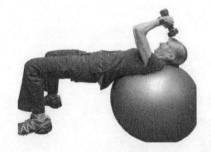

the TheraBand brand, because of its resistance and durability.

TheraBand makes a great exercise ball that can be used for many years, as long the dog doesn't chew on it or a spouse puts it in the garage: the two most common excuses for not using the ball at home.

Unstable Surfaces & Lower Back Pain
A 2010 study published in the *Journal of Orthopedic and Sports Physical Therapy* titled, "Trunk Muscle Activity During Lumbar Stabilization Exercises on Both a Stable and Unstable Surface," evaluated how core muscles were activated on unstable and stable surfaces. Unstable surfaces challenged the lower back and core muscles more than when the exercises were performed on the ground.
https://www.ncbi.nlm.nih.gov/pubmed/20511695

Unstable surfaces make almost every exercise more difficult and enhance neuromuscular training. The exercises do not have to be extremely difficult; they simply make the stabilizer muscles work harder than a person is used to: the reason unstable surface exercises enhance low back recovery.

In the gym, BOSU balls and foam pads are unstable surfaces that make exercises more challenging. I do not recommend patients purchasing a BOSU ball for home use because it has fewer applications and the inexpensive ones are not built well. Foam pads can be used for many types of exercises and take up less space.

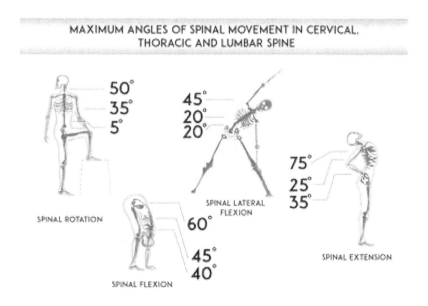

It Sounded Good. Why Wouldn't It Be the Best Course of Action?

At 19 I was working at a golf course when a heavy week of rain had put us behind in mowing, and the biggest tournament of the year was three days away. The boss's wife graciously volunteered to help us out by helping mow the fairways.

I was in charge of training Maria on how to use the mower. I went through the process and procedure of how to run the mower and activate the cutting reels. At the last second I decided to tell her that the mower does not turn right, it only makes left-hand turns. I explained that turning right could create an electrical problem and short the mower. "We don't have time to fix it correctly, so please only make left-hand turns."

To my advantage, it did sound like something her husband would rig up with his patch work mechanical skills, combining duct tape and wire, and it did fall under his "customized" category.

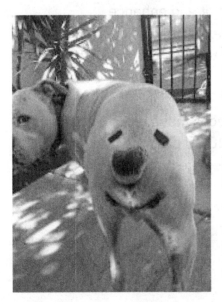

I walked back up to the club house with a big grin on my face. The boss saw my look and knew I was up to something, looking down the hill he started laughing. He saw her making a wide, left-turning loop when a sharper right U-turn would have been more efficient. Then on the other side she made the proper right U-turn. All he said was, "you are in so much trouble when she finds out." Needless to say, it took her longer than it should have to mow the fairway and she never volunteered to help again. She did get me back a couple years later, with the help of her old high school classmate Police Officer Johnson.

It was my job to provide her with the best instruction possible, and anything less was a failure on my part. She believed me to be the expert and didn't question my instructions. It sounded reasonable. She didn't have any reason to suspect I was not giving her the most efficient and effective instructions.

In the office we hear many stories from patients who liked their provider and thought he or she did a great job. They never realized that they were getting the wrong instructions for the job. The information might have gotten the job done, but was not the best or most efficient way to accomplish the task. These patients were basically trying to mow the fairway by only taking left-hand turns.

I do not think that the other providers are intentionally giving bad advice. I just believe that it is their job to be the best teacher and provider possible, and there is no room for below-average in healthcare. Nobody likes having his or her time wasted or being ineffective because of bad advice. Therefore, if one provider cannot figure out the most effective path for improving your back pain, go get help from someone else before considering surgery.

We work hard to give you the best treatment and advice possible. There is more than one way to "mow a fairway," and we strive for the most efficient path possible. I like to think that our office is pretty good, has plenty of treatment options, and works hard for patients. But we can't help everyone.

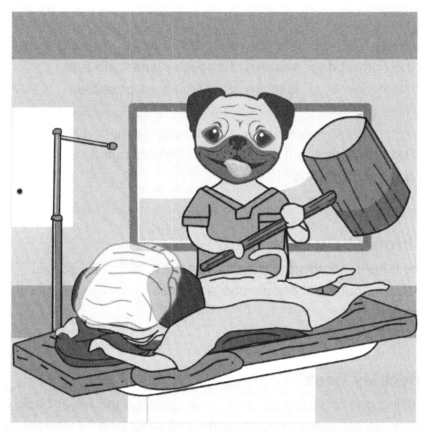

For patients with continued chronic localized low back pain, we will refer to another conservative treatment provider before surgery. A treatment trial with another facility is always worth it. If the problem persists, the patient can feel better that he or she tried everything possible before bringing the "biggest hammer" to the back problems.

Low back surgery can be effective for some people, while for others it creates a different series of problems. We never know who will have good results and who will have problems, so make the decision to go forward after significant thought, research, and effort with conservative treatments.

Surgery is bringing the "biggest hammer" to your low back. There is no way to undo this hammer swing, so swing it wisely.

Chapter 26: Common Surgery Questions

Does My Past Back Surgery Mean I Will Always Have Pain?
Most times people can return to a higher level of function and hopefully pain-free activity. Every surgery and every patient is different; do not listen to your friends about their experience and make comparisons regarding your own condition.

Surgery can be minimally invasive: i.e. pulling a disc extrusion away from a nerve root. A more complicated surgery might involve inserting multiple plates and screws, which will permanently alter back function.

My feeling is that after back surgery, your job is to get your back in as good shape as is possible. We cannot change the current degenerative changes or wear-and-tear injuries. However, we *can* make the low back function as optimally as possible.

Depending on degeneration, age, strength, endurance, and core function, certain activities will need to be modified or avoided, but most people can continue a very active lifestyle without fear of additional surgery.

Do I Need Surgery for Chronic Low Back Pain?
No. Most people never require surgery for low back pain. There are definitely some instances that require it immediately, but most people can wait to see how they respond to quality conservative treatment.

Would Knee Surgery Affect My Back?
Any surgery that alters the walking gait can produce excessive strain on the lower back. Hip and knee replacement surgeries are very common today, and most people improve significantly after those surgeries. Unfortunately, some people do not reach optimal levels and end up with an altered gait. Some lose the ability to squat, creating excessive low back strain due to hinging when bending forward.

The low back, hips, knees, ankles, and feet work together as a system to walk, bend, twist, or participate in sports. Limitation in any of the lower extremity joints can increase strain in the lower back, resulting in future back injuries.

What Symptoms Require Back Surgery?

Loss of bowel and bladder control requires immediate surgical intervention. Back surgery should be considered for lumbar disc extrusions that severely compress the spinal cord or nerve roots and create neurologic conditions, such as loss of motor strength, reflexes, or sensation. Foot drop is a significant sign of severe nerve compression.

Is Surgery Effective for Disc Extrusions?

Multiple types of surgery are effective at grabbing a disc extrusion and pulling it out of the spinal cord, reducing compression on the nerves. A large disc extrusion could take years to be dissolved by the body, and a surgical removal is many times the best solution.

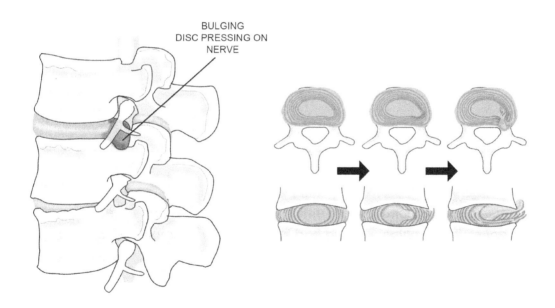

For example, I have had patients with a large disc extrusion compressing nerve roots and experiencing severe pain. Treatments provided short periods of relief, but back and leg pain returned within a few hours. They spent more time trying to minimize their pain than doing anything else in their lives.

I don't think it is worth it to suffer for six months or more to avoid surgery, especially since surgery will immediately relieve their pain. My feeling is to remove the source of pain, and then spend the next few months making sure it won't happen again through proper rehabilitation.

I do believe people need to be informed about their type of surgery, risks, spinal consequences, and expectations for the future. Too many times I see people jump into surgery because of the short term pain, and not understand their options.

Does Lower Back Surgery Work?
Yes, surgery can be fantastic and dramatically improve a person's life. When a surgeon removes a disc herniation that is compressing the nerve root, leg pain is dramatically reduced. But it doesn't eliminate the spinal stabilization issue that led to pain in the first place.

Surgery has a purpose. It can be a part of a person's treatment, but it shouldn't be the only treatment. People who think that surgery is going to eliminate future risks are fooling themselves.

Imagine that your car needs an alignment and has four older tires. If one tire gets a nail hole and leaks, you can patch that tire to restore tire pressure. Patching the tire solved the air leak problem, but it did not make the car track properly.

Getting an alignment will improve tracking; however, it cannot fix the wear on the tires. A well-aligned car will get more miles out of the tires, but expectations need to be managed.

Low back surgery is tremendous for removing the disc extrusion to reduce radiating pain. Rehabilitation involves aligning and stabilizing spinal movements for long-term performance.

What Is Successful Disc Surgery?
A successful disc surgery is defined as removing the extrusion, patching up the disc, removing the nerve compression, and eliminating radicular pain. The surgery will not fix damage to the facet joints, injuries above and below the disc extrusion, nor will it restore muscular spinal stabilization. It does not remove all of the pain sources in the lower back, nor does it prevent future outbreaks of pain.

Increasing Risks of Lumbar Fusion After Discectomy

A March 2019 study published in the *Spine Journal* titled, "Lumbar Discectomy is Associated with Higher Rates of Lumbar Fusion," stated that patients who undergo disectomy are three times more likely to undergo lumbar spinal fusion within 10 years compared to those who did not undergo the surgery.

A patient who chooses not to undergo lumbar discectomy has a 4.19-percent change of undergoing spinal fusion compared to 12.5 percent for those who had the discectomy at 10 years. https://www.ncbi.nlm.nih.gov/pubmed/29792995

Risks After Discectomy for Another Disc Herniation

In a 2018 study published in the *Journal of Bone and Joint Surgery* titled, "Patients at the HIghest Risk for Re Herniation Following Lumbar Discectomy in a Multicenter Randomized Controlled Trial," researchers found that after two years, there was a 25-percent likelihood of recurrence when the annular disc tear was between 6-10mm wide by 4-6mm long. The average second herniation was 264 days following surgery, and over half of those patients had a second surgery.
https://www.ncbi.nlm.nih.gov/pmc/articles/PMC6145569/#

Larger disc injuries carry a greater risk of second herniation within two years of surgery. Patients who have disc injuries in this range need to pay extra attention to their rehabilitation and restrictions after discectomy to avoid additional injuries.

Will Surgery Solve My Back Pain?

A 2015 study published by *Clinical Orthopedics and Related Research* titled, "Incidence of Low Back Pain After Lumbar Discectomy for Herniated Disc and Its Effect on Patient reported Outcomes," stated that between four percent and 34 percent of patients will report short term or chronic back pain two years after surgery. The two-year incidence of a second herniation ranged from zero percent to 23 percent and frequency of reoperation between zero to 13 percent.
https://www.ncbi.nlm.nih.gov/pubmed/25694267

This was a systematic study combining results from multiple resources, hence the wide range of results. Even with the range it does confirm other studies showing that between 20 and 30 percent of people will have chronic back pain two years after surgery, and that the risk of a second surgery is around 10 percent within two years of the first surgery.

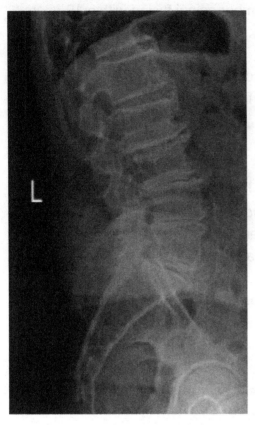

Leg Pain After Surgery?
Radiating leg pain should disappear after surgery. In severe cases it may take the nerve time to heal and repair, especially after damage from severe nerve root compressions.

Pain in the middle of the back may or may not disappear. It depends on how much of the pain was from the compression. If the middle back pain is caused by joints and ligaments, that pain will continue but can be improved with physical therapy.

Bones Spurs and Surgery?
When the surgeon needs to remove degenerative bone spurs in order to widen the space for the exiting nerve, the surgery is more involved. Patients must understand that the complexity of surgery and recovery times increase with every location the surgeon modifies.

At the end of the day, a very small nerve root hole is bad, and a bigger hole is better. You reduced the opening size through poor spinal movement that led to the degeneration. Focus on rehab to slow continued degeneration in the area.

How Long Will It Take To Recover From Surgery?
It depends on the problem and the type of surgery. With minimally invasive surgeries, recovery could be a few weeks, while more invasive procedures could take months. Don't listen to your friends' experience on this one. Ask the surgeon and staff what is involved, and how long the restrictions are in place.

Specifically ask them how long before you can golf, run, or perform any activity you want, and then add 25-50 percent more time for an average recovery.

How Serious Is Back Surgery?

Lower back surgery does have risks, as with any surgical procedure. The less involved the surgery, the fewer the risks. When plates and screws are added, the risks increase. Be informed and ask multiple providers for their thoughts and recommendations.

When the conservation turns to adding hardware, my rule of thumb is exhaust every other treatment option first. Do not jump to surgery without several months of good rehab.

Fusing spinal levels does increase disc space, but it does not fix the facet degeneration problem. It will also cause increased stress loads above and below the fusion level that may lead to problems in the future.

It could be a robbing-Peter-to-pay-Paul situation, especially if you do not work hard in the rehabilitation phase.

Spinal fusion could also be a critical step in your recovery. Try everything else first to make sure it is necessary, then work hard on core stabilization to prevent future problems.

Surgeries Gone Wrong

As mentioned before, every surgery has risks. Every provider has examples of fusion surgeries that have gone extremely well, but they also have cases in which it has gone horribly wrong. Infections are always a risk, and when they occur, they are devastating. One failed surgery can quickly lead to a second or third.

Be informed about the procedure. A person has to accept the risk and be ready for the unfavorable result once he or she chooses invasive surgery.

I never recommend jumping to invasive surgery to fix severe pain. These are the instances when patients are the least happy with their outcomes.

Why Does One of My Friends Still Have Problems After Surgery?

I do not know the specifics of your friend or their specific problem. Generally when I see patients who are not happy with their back surgery, it is because they expected the procedure to completely fix the problem or they didn't reach their therapeutic rehabilitation goals.

Sometimes it comes from a surgeon who tells the patient he or she doesn't need rehab after surgery because the problem was fixed. The surgeon believes everything is a structural problem and completely ignores the movement components and functions. These are my least favorite surgeons. They completely ignore *how* the patient ended up with this damage and what is *best for long term recovery*.

Not going through rehab after surgery only works for those athletic individuals, in excellent condition, and without degenerative changes. Think of the 20-30-year-old athlete, not a person who can live in an age-restricted community.

Let's go back to the car. Patching the tire and not getting an alignment works for newer tires that are well aligned, not for tires with lots of miles on them.

In addition to spinal stabilization and strengthening exercises, aerobic exercises have been found to enhance recovery from single level-disc surgeries. *The European Journal of Physical and Rehabilitation Medicine* published an article in 2010 evaluating improvement using aerobic exercise one month after surgery. The article titled, "The Effects of Early Aerobic Exercise After Single Level Lumbar Microdiscectomy: a Prospective, Controlled Trial," showed that aerobic exercise improved functional abilities post surgery.

My personal bias is that every individual with chronic low back pain presents with a specific compensation and guarding mechanism. Proper rehabilitation helps to activate dysfunctional muscles, to restore spinal stability and enhance function. Multiple activities can activate these muscles, but correct exercises need to be given to restore proper function. https://www.ncbi.nlm.nih.gov/pubmed/20935605

Why Is My Other Friend Happy with Surgery?

For some people surgery is a very good option, and the procedure and rehabilitation go well. There are many people who are very happy with their lower back surgeries. It is easy to pick on the failed surgeries, but it is important to acknowledge the critical role surgery plays in people's lives when it comes to solving structural back problems.

A 2007 study published in the *European Spine Journal*, "Early Neuromuscular Customized Training After Surgery or Lumbar Disc Herniation: a Prospective Controlled

Study," compared traditional physical therapy after surgery to early integration of neuromuscular training after lumbar disc herniation surgery. The early neuromuscular group showed significant improvement over traditional therapy with regard to pain and function. https://www.ncbi.nlm.nih.gov/pmc/articles/PMC2198880/

The study demonstrates the benefits of early therapy that emphasizes muscle patterns and neuromuscular control following surgery. The low back is not ready for heavy exercises; however, it shows significant benefit from muscle activation exercises.

Can I Get a Hernia After Back Surgery?

The surgery did not cause the hernia. The poor muscular system combined with previous wear and tear led to the hernia. Think of it this way: hernias are more likely to occur when a person does not have good core and pelvic muscular stabilization. These are the same factors that lead to spinal degeneration and disc injuries.

Usually a person is compromised for a few months leading up to surgery, which increases tissue strain. After surgery, the muscles are not immediately activated or strong. It takes time and work to restore proper muscle function. Unfortunately, the tissue damage can be cumulative and a hernia develops during the recovery stage.

Knee Pain After Surgery?

A compromised lower back changes the way a person uses his/her hips and knees to walk and bend. The increased strain from the body trying to protect the back leads to injuries elsewhere. Most of these injuries are to the muscles, tendons, and ligaments around joints, as opposed to structural damage to the meniscus or bone.

During post-surgical rehabilitation, evaluation of your movement patterns, walking gait, and lower extremity mechanics will address weaknesses and future risk factors. We find that many people with low back pain have compromised knee function due to years of low back guarding and compensating.

We make it a point to prescribe exercises that improve knee stability, flexibility, and strength for every low back patient. There are many exercises that enhance how the lower extremities work with the back to transfer power and reduce strain on the lumbar spine.

Video: How to Avoid Back Surgery

Chapter 27: Low Back Exercises

Acute lower back pain can happen with a sudden movement, twist, bending motion, or lifting activity. People can either experience a sharp, stabbing pain right when they injure their lower back, or they can feel it slowly progress over time. Sometimes the pain can increase for 1 to 2 days before becoming severe and limiting.

During the acute phase, our goals are to decrease pain, muscle spasms, and inflammation in an injured area. This is not the time to be aggressive with the injury. You are essentially going downhill, and our goals are to stop the dissent and get you going in the right direction. Ice is an excellent treatment during this time. It does a tremendous job of decreasing pain and inflammation.

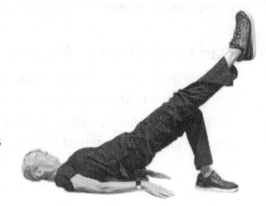

Light movement exercises can be performed to decrease pain. Joint movement blocks pain sensors from sending signals to the brain. Light movement also tells the body that it is okay and not as injured is it may think. All exercises should be performed in a pain-free range of motion. If it hurts, stop! Don't go that far. All exercises should be a nice, slow, and controlled rock in a pain-free zone.

After several repetitions. you might find an increased ability to move further without pain. This is not the time to push your luck.

Sometimes people think that if some is good, more is better. This is not the case with acute injuries. Remember, you are going downhill after injuring a muscle, tendon, or joint. Trying to push too hard during the acute phase increases the possibility of exacerbating your injury or increasing your muscle spasms.

All low back exercises with pictures, description, and videos can be found at:
http://www.robertsonfamilychiro.com/low_back_exercise_video_series_chandler_az.htm

Be smart and reasonable while reducing future injury risks,

Alpha Chiropractic & Physical Therapy
www.robertsonfamilychiro.com
(480) 812-1800

Acute Pain and Range of Motion Exercises
Light and easy exercises to reduce pain and daily sourness.

Knee Side-to-Side
Perform the knee side-to-side exercises in a slow and controlled manner. Start on your back with your knees bent. Very slowly rock them to your left, stopping before experiencing any pain or spasms. Slowly rock back to a neutral position and toward the right, once again stopping if you experience any lower back pain. Slowly rock your knees back and forth 15 to 20 times.

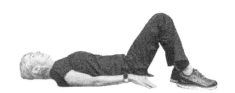

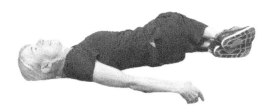
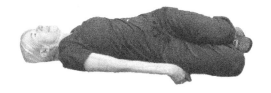

Knee to Chest
Laying on your back with knees bent, grab your right knee with both hands and pull it toward the chest. You should feel a comfortable stretch. Hold for 20 seconds, then release the stretch for a few seconds and stretch toward the chest again. Repeat with the other leg. If those go well, pull both knees to the chest for a comfortable stretch. For a greater stretch, pull one knee to the chest and straighten the other leg.

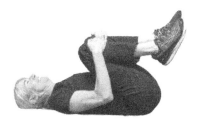
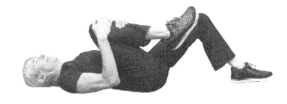

Review of Knee Side-to-Side and Knee to Chest:

Pelvic Tilts

Pelvic tilt exercises can also be performed if the first two are going well. Either in a sitting or lying position, tip your pelvis forward, pausing for a few seconds before tipping your pelvis backwards. Slowly tip your pelvis forward with a pause before rocking backwards. Repeat this 15 to 20 times.

I like to describe these exercises as rusty door hinge exercises. Slowly rock the back joints to increase movement, just as if you were trying to rock a rusty door hinge gate. With a rusty hinge, there is not any advantage to being overly aggressive and kicking the gate open. It is better to be slow and safe in order to decrease pain and reduce the risk of further damage.

Cat / Camel / Child's Pose

The back can be stretched in camel (image 1), cat (image 2), and child's pose (image 3) positions. Twisting and turning the torso can cause a stretch from the warrior pose or kneeling lunges. On your hands and knees, lower your stomach to the ground for camel. Then pull the stomach up toward the spine and round the back for cat position. For child's pose, lean the waist backwards while keeping the hands on the table. A light stretch should be felt in the low back.

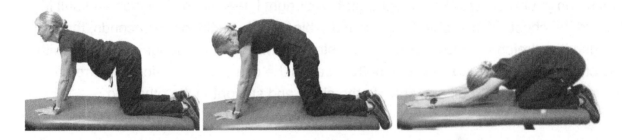

Hip Stretch

Another exercise you can perform while lying on your back is to pull your left knee toward your chin. You should experience a light, comfortable stretch in your lower back and hip muscles. Stop if it hurts.

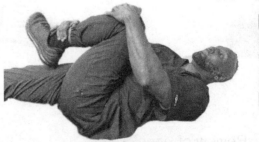

After holding for a few seconds, slowly pull your left knee toward your right shoulder. Then pull toward your right elbow. Each position will stretch a different part of the hip. Repeat the raising and lowering of the left knee 10 times. This exercise can then be repeated on the right side. For increasing stretch pull on the ankle and rotate the leg.

The pigeon pose in yoga can be modified by using a bench. Place the crossed leg on the bench at 90 degrees and then lean forward with your torso. Reaching to the left or right will change the stretch.

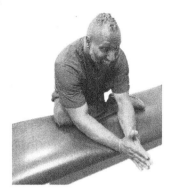
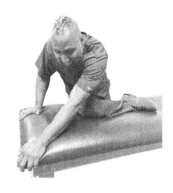

Thoracic Rotation

Twisting and rotating can stretch the hip and low back. Changing the torso angle and knee position changes the stretch. The sitting version is shown in image 1 by crossing the left leg over the right. Take the right arm and reach toward the left. A stronger variation is to pull the right elbow into the left knee to enhance the rotation. Image 2 and 3 show the rotation variations in the lunge stretch series that also stretch the low back. A standing version using the wall for support with explanation can be found by watching the video.

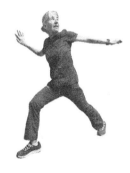
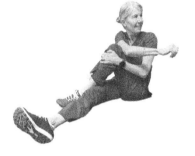
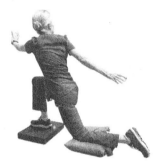

Cobra

Cobra position can stretch the back into extension by keeping the waist on the ground. The easiest stretch is to extend the torso backwards by pressing onto the forearms. A stronger variation is to extend backwards by pushing from your hands. *Do not force the extension movements, especially with a prior history of low back pain.

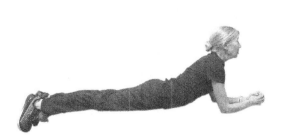
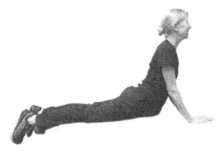

Stretching With the Stick

Use a stick or broom handle to help you stretch. One hand can help push the other into a comfortable stretch, obtaining more range of motion than without the assistance. With two hands on the stick, raise both arms above the head and stretch as far as comfortably possible (image 1). With the stick above your head, laterally bend to the side (image 2), and repeat to the other side. Image 3 shows how the right hand can be stretched further into extension by pushing the stick with the left hand. Lowering the right hand 45 degrees and extending backwards with the side of the left hand pushing will enhance the chest and shoulder stretch (image 4).

The next position is lowering the arm another 45 degrees and stretching the shoulder without rotating the body. Image 5 shows this stretch for the left shoulder. Image 6 shows the same stretch with the addition of thoracic rotation.

Any of the stretches can be modified with thoracic rotation or extension. Often people benefit by doing the stretch with the torso in neutral position and then stretching a second time with the torso rotated. Stay comfortable and do not force the positions or stretches; all should be performed pain free.

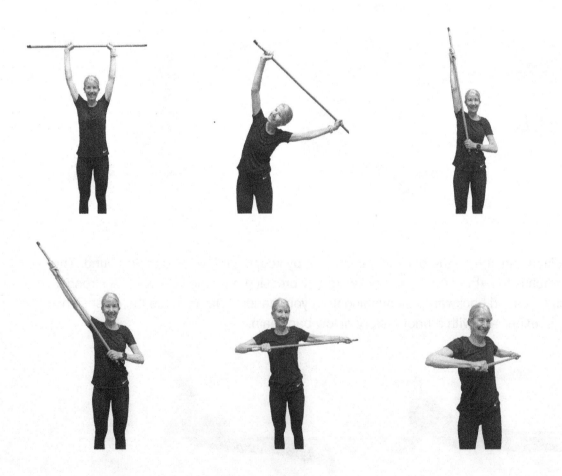

Lower Leg

The calf stretch can be performed standing with the foot flat on the ground, on a step, or with a foot rocker (prostretch). Having the knee straight or bent will focus the stretch on the two different calf muscles: gastrocnemius and soleus.

Place the left foot behind you with the heel on the ground. Glide your waist and body weight forward until a stretch is felt in the calf (image 1). Hold onto a wall for extra support if needed. Performing the same stretch with a bent knee will focus more of the stretch onto the soleus muscle.

Using a prostretch or calf rocker is another variation. Place your right foot onto the rocker and push the heel toward the floor. Watch the Calf Stretch with Pro Stretch explanation.

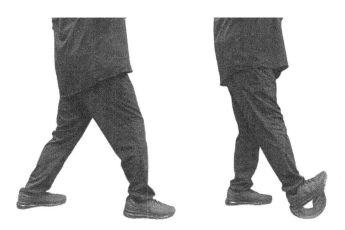

The front of the lower leg can be stretched by either pulling your ankle backwards or resting it on a bench with the toe pointed (image 1). Sitting on the heel will create a greater stretch (image 2).

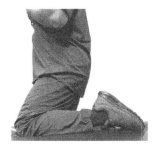
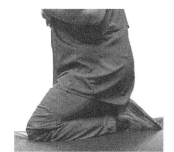

Lunge Series

Forward Lunge

Start with your arms at your sides. If you feel unsteady, do this exercise near a wall, table or sturdy chair to hold onto. Lunge forward with one leg. Glide the waist forward and slightly lower until a stretch is felt. As with squats, it is not necessary to do a full, deep lunge to benefit from this exercise. Move the forward leg back to the starting position and lunge forward with the opposite leg. Start with one set of 10 and work your way up to two sets (image 1).

Initially, do not lower your waist all the way to the ground. Perform the exercise in a stable and controlled manner. With increased leg and hip strength, you will be able to go lower and perform more repetitions. A variation is to raise the opposite arm in the air and extend the torso backwards (image 2). Another option is to rotate the torso and arm (image 3). Do not force or strain with the torso or arm variations.

To make it easier, the lunge can be performed with a knee on the ground for stability. A pillow or towel can be placed under the knees for comfort (images 4, 5, and 6).

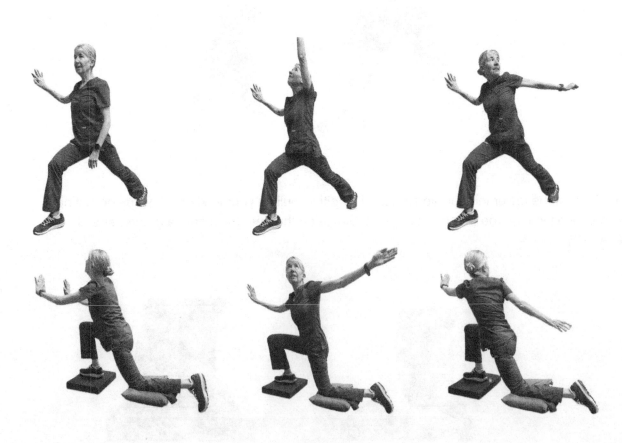

Side Lunge & Adductors

With two feet wide apart, lean with the waist to the left. A stretch should be felt on the inside of the upper leg or groin area. The stretch can be changed by pointing the foot straight, inward, or outward. Repeat both sides.

The adductors can be stretched in the standing lunge position or the butterfly stretch. Pushing into the knees increases the stretch; likewise, leaning forward can also increase the stretch.

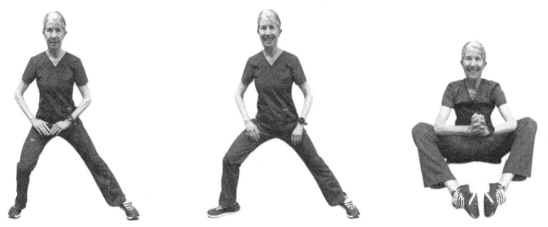

Hamstrings & Adductors

Hamstrings can be stretched standing or sitting. The long hamstring muscles run on the inside and outside of the back of the leg. Turning the toe in or out will change the muscle group getting stretched. Having the legs together or apart also changes the stretch. Bend your knees to change the region of the hamstrings getting stretched. Try a little in every position.

A rope or strap can also be used to increase the forward torso pull, especially if you cannot reach your feet.

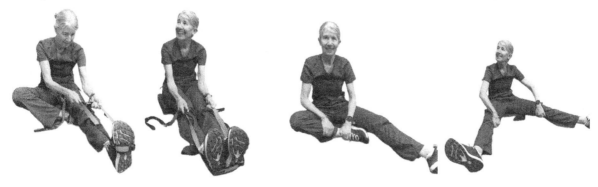

Quadriceps & Hip Flexors with Table

A table or bench can enhance a quadriceps and hip flexor stretch. Using the floor or bench, step forward with one leg and leave the other lagging behind. The further the legs are apart, the greater the hip flexor stretch. Twisting the hips to the left or right will change the hip flexor stretch.

The closer the foot gets to the glutes, the greater the quadriceps stretch (image 2). Grab the foot or use a rope to provide a greater stretch. (Image 3)

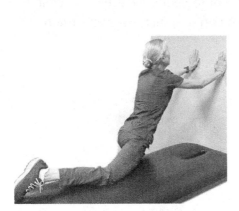
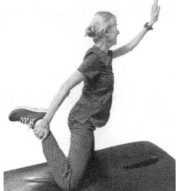
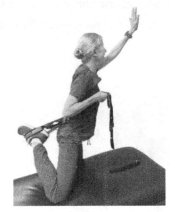

Pulling the ankle inward (image 1), straight (image 2) , or outward (image 3) will change the quadriceps stretch. The examples below are showing the quadriceps being stretched while laying on your stomach. Pulling the foot in different directions will help stretch all the parts of the quadriceps muscles.

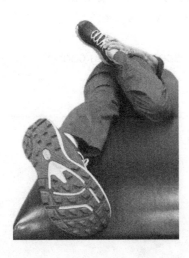
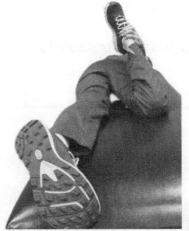
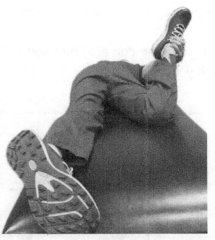

Sub Basement Exercises

Knee flexion and extension
Start with the knee bent and hanging off a chair, table or bench. Slowly extend the knee. Pause at full extension and flex the knee as far as comfortably possible. The exercise can be made more difficult by adding an ankle weight or resistance rubber band.

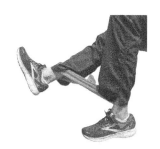

Seated hip abduction and adduction
Abduction is taking your upper leg to the side, and adduction brings the leg back to the middle. Initially the exercises can be performed in a chair, but you should quickly advance to a lying or standing position. Once again, the exercises can be made more difficult by adding a resistance band.

Seated hip Internal and external rotation
Internal hip rotation is when the femur and knee turns inward, and external rotation is the opposite motion. In a seated position with your knees bent at a 90-degree angle, place your right foot on the ground and lift the right ankle across the left. Try to keep the femur in the same position while pivoting the ankle. Repeat this motion 10 times, then the opposite motion. By anchoring the rubber resistance band to the bottom of the chair and ankle, the band will apply resistance throughout the motions.

From seated positions we move to standing. We always want to master the simpler exercise before progressing to harder exercises. Challenging the body's proprioception (balance) system increases your neurologic learning and accelerates your recovery.

The exercises always start with your eyes open. When you feel fairly steady, close one eye. This causes a loss of depth perception. Closing both eyes is significantly harder.

Always perform eyes closed exercises in a safe environment when you can grab onto something for support, such as a wall or cane.

Base-Level Standing Exercises to Develop Proprioception

Nobody likes working on exercises they are not very good at. We all want to work on things that we enjoy and feel that we do a great job with. Many of the exercises and stability work are difficult and challenge your system. *It challenges all of the things you are not very good at, for a very good reason.* You have balance issues because the system is compromised.

Over time you will notice improvement in your ability to perform these exercises. You will be able to do them longer and with better control. Eventually you will fatigue, but it will take longer to hit your failure point. **That is an improvement.**

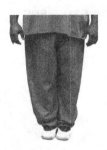 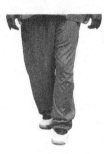 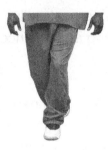 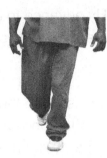 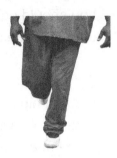

Together   **Modified Tandem**   **Tandem**   **Single leg toe down**   **Single leg**

The simplest of standing exercises is tandem stance, where you have one foot in front of the other like you're walking on a tightrope. For many people this is the initial exercise that they can properly perform. If you're having weakness and feel like you can't stay balanced in this position, then that's a sign of significant proprioceptive loss.

To make this exercise a step harder, close one eye. At this point we're losing input from our eyes, which helps with our stability. By losing a little bit of depth perception, it requires your body to listen to the ankle, knee, and hip joint receptors to keep stable.

Many people become very eye dominant for their proprioception. They stopped listening to their foot, ankle, knee, and hip joint receptors. For long term improvement, you need to reactivate the joint proprioceptors. Closing both eyes makes the exercise much harder and is one of the fastest ways to engage this system and enhance your recovery (be safe when and where you close your eyes - no falling).

From the tandem stance we can progress to a single leg stance with the knee slightly bent. We want to maintain proper posture in the back and hips, which then require the lower leg, upper leg, hip, and back muscles to work together. Single leg stance is making several muscular and nervous systems work together. This may sound simple, but I think you should try it before reading the next paragraph.

Rule of Thumb:
You should be able to hold your single leg stance position for over a minute with your eyes closed.

Try standing on one foot and squatting. If you can't stand on one foot try it with two feet shoulder width apart. As you lower yourself, you'll notice that at some point you will want to hinge forward. <u>The point of the hinge is a sign of your strength levels.</u>

You were probably only able to squat another six to eight inches before hinging forward. <u>This is your breaking point</u>. Past this point you are unable to stabilize the knee, pelvis, or back because of muscle weakness. Your body went to its usual compensation method of hinging forward: lowering your shoulders towards the ground without moving your hips anymore. And yes, you should be able to squat lower on one leg then you just did for this test.

Further enhancement of the proprioceptive system involves unstable surfaces. There are a variety of unstable services that can be utilized. Anything soft and squishy, such as foam or rubber discs, works well. From here we can progress to more unstable services such as a wooden wobble or rocker board. Many people are familiar with BOSU balls, which have a rubber dome on one side and a flat, hard plastic side on the reverse. We can stand on both the rubber or hard plastic, and each have a different level of difficulty and enhance activation of muscle stabilizers (Journal of Strength Conditioning and Research).

Each of these exercises can be enhanced by closing one or both eyes. The more you require the body and brain to listen to the joint sensors in the ankle, knee, and foot, the faster you will improve.

All of these neuromuscular pattern exercises can be enhanced with a vibration unit. Vibration units continually knock you off balance, which requires the system to pull you back to neutral and stabilize. In the meantime you have been shifting to the opposite direction again and your body has to respond. The speed, amplitude, and frequency of vibration can be adjusted and each has a therapeutic advantage.

Rule of Thumb:

<u>Stimulus and Response.</u> The body responds to changing stimuli. If you want a reaction or different outcome, you need to challenge the body. The more stimulus we challenge you with, the faster you will respond. This is why level one exercises are great at the beginning but you need to progress past these to more challenging exercises.

Exercise balls can be utilized in many of the following exercises. Balance is more than just your feet and ankles. The pelvis, core, and back play an integral role in maintaining balance as you stand and walk.

Sitting on a ball makes the pelvis and core work together to keep steady. Adding arm movements or weights challenges the system even more. The exercises are always made easier with a wide base, two feet apart. Moving the feet closer together changes your stability and makes the body work harder. Eventually you can perform the same exercise with two feet tandem or on a single leg..

Most people are amazed at how difficult it is to maintain balance on a vibration plate. Every exercise is significantly harder and more challenging, which speeds your overall neuromuscular control and recovery.

Training on a vibration therapy machine is an excellent way to increase proprioception, blood flow, muscle strength, endurance, and stimulate muscle growth. The increased level of difficulty and entire body muscle contraction increases the effort and calories burned per hour, which can result in increased weight loss compared to performing the same exercises on the ground.

Our office utilizes vibration machines to quickly and efficiently develop neuromuscular patterns, strength, and endurance in injured areas.

Vibration, Unstable Surfaces, and Proprioception

Vibration plates have been around for many years and are used by all advanced or high-tech rehabilitation or sports training facilities. Athletes can utilize vibration therapy to further develop their proprioceptive sensors, enhancing their stability and neuromuscular control. Even a person who is in great shape can find vibration therapy difficult.

It's all about challenging the system and getting the body to respond. Every individual has his breaking point, and as a provider it is my job to identify your weakness and move you past it. We have had exceptional athletes get even better while challenging their one leg squat with their eyes closed. Of course they usually squat much lower and require more repetitions to reach their weakness. But the theory and process are the same.

The Exercise Progression
We always want to master the simpler exercise before progressing to harder exercises. Challenging the body's proprioception (balance) system increases your neurologic learning and accelerates your recovery.

The exercises always start with your eyes open. When you feel fairly steady, close one eye. This causes a loss of depth perception. Closing both eyes is significantly harder. Always perform eyes closed exercises in a safe environment when you can grab onto something for support, such as a wall or cane.

Challenge but don't overwhelm

This is a simple rule for balance exercises. Challenge the system but don't overwhelm. If your activity is overwhelming the body then it is not learning or adapting. The greatest improvement always comes with challenging your abilities with slightly harder exercises to make the system learn. The body does not learn when it is overwhelmed.

A long time ago I could stand on an exercise ball.

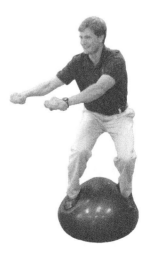

Basement Low Back Exercises

Sometimes you have to start in the basement and that is ok. It is not where you start, it is where you end.

Door Frame Series

The Door Frame series works to improve balance, along with how well the lower extremity works with the pelvis and core. In a door frame, start with two feet together. Keep your hands near the door frame to touch for support. Close one eye and try to keep steady, open the eye as needed or touch the door frame. With improvement close both eyes and maintain balance.

With improvement you can make the exercise more challenging by moving one foot backwards to a modified tandem position. The next hardest position is having the feet right behind each other, as if you were walking a tightrope. In each of these positions plastic having both eyes open, one eye closed, and both eyes closed. No falling!

Single leg stance

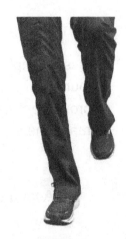

Stand on one foot and stay steady. Your eyes and head should be facing forward with the shoulders and waist aligned. The knee should be pointing straight forward and not rocking inward. Your body weight should be distributed across the middle of your standing foot, while the foot arch is maintained and not flattening inward.

To make the exercises even harder, you can add slow squats or weights to the exercises. The exercises can also be performed on increasing unstable surfaces, such as a folded up towel, foam, BOSU ball, rocker board, wobble board, or vibration plate.

All of the exercises start on the ground and then progress to a more unstable surface.

Door Frame Rotational Exercises

With the same foot positions as the door frame series this exercise will add rotation. Take the right hand and reach toward the left door frame. Try to hold the hand just above the frame without touching. Then slowly reach with the left hand toward the right door frame, focusing on slow rotation of the torso while maintaining balance. As in the door frame exercise, start with two feet together and then progress to tandem or single leg position. It is easier with both eyes open and then make the exercise harder by closing one eye. With improvement try closing both eyes and slowly rotating to the door frames.

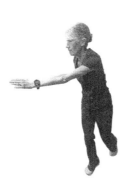 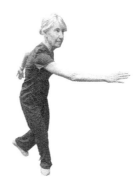

Standing Hip Exercises: Door Frame (45° / 90°/ 180°)
Standing hip exercises challenge the hip stabilizer while incorporating balance activities. We begin the exercise inside a door frame for stability by keeping our hands on the frame, and with improvement taking the hands off. The exercises incorporate three planes of movement. The exercise takes the leg to the side, backwards, and at a 45 degree angle.

The three positions work all of the glute muscles; max, medius, and minimus muscles while incorporating balance and pelvic stability. With improvement an exercise band can be added to make the exercise more difficult

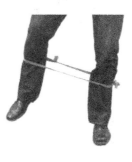

Calf raises

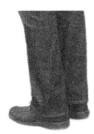 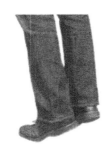

Standing with two feet shoulder width apart, slowly raise your heels off the ground as you keep your balance. Then slowly lower your heels back to the ground. Initially start with two feet, then progress to single leg when your strength improves.

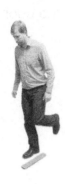
Side steps foam
Start by standing on your right leg with the left held slightly above the ground. Step to the left and shift weight to the left leg. Then lean back to the right and raise your left foot off the ground. Once you are steady on your right leg, repeat the exercise 10 times per side.

Step ups
Start with a three-inch aerobics step. Stand behind the step and practice stepping forward and up the step while keeping your knee pointing forward. Try not to shift your body weight to the side, compensating for hip and knee weakness. Over time and improvement, increase the height of the step. Increase stride length to add difficulty.

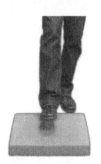

Modified plank
You can do a modified plank exercise off the side of your bed or a sturdy table. Position your arms on the table or bed so that they are directly below your shoulders. You may want to grasp your hands together to be more stable. Now move your feet straight out behind you. Imagine a straight line that connects your head, shoulders, hips and feet. That is the perfect plank. Start by holding this position for 10-15 seconds and work your way up to sixty seconds.

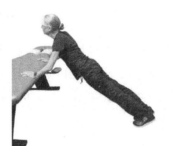

Modified push-up
The difference between a modified push up and a full military push up is that you pivot from your knees as opposed to your feet. You can also do full push ups off of a wall, or an incline push up off of a bench using the modified position.

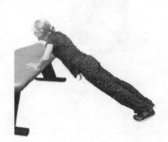

Plank From Knees
Planks are a tremendous exercise for increasing rectus abdominis and oblique muscle strength, which is commonly lost in people with chronic knee pain. Plank exercises can be modified by starting on your knees instead of feet, which makes the exercise significantly easier. Start where you can and then progress as you are able. People with back pain and weakness increase strain on their knees. Getting the core stronger will reduce some of your knee pain.

Sit to Stand
Getting out of a chair requires hip and leg strength. There are ways to increase hip and quadriceps strength by using the chair. We can keep our feet two feet apart and place our hands on our knees to help push and stabilize. A second step is to move the feet closer together. With improvement push off your leg with less force. The feet can also be staggered for the sit to stand.

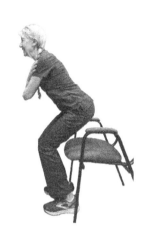

Another way to build strength is from a standing position, try and lower yourself to the chair without using your hands. You will feel yourself "plunk down" on the table. This is the point where the hip strength was unable to support the body.

Seated leg-raise
Sit on the ball with your arms crossed or by your side. Slowly raise the left leg, lower it and then raise the right leg. Repeat ten times with each leg for a set. Eventually you can add a weight to hold in front of you or to the side for added difficulty.

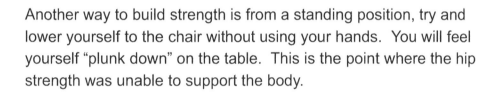

FlexBar Shake
Do this exercise while sitting on an exercise ball or standing. Hold one end of the FlexBar and extend your arm out to the side or out in front. Then shake the bar. This exercise will enhance your grip, upper arm, and shoulder strength. To make things more challenging, do woodchopper movements while shaking the Flexbar. Twisting at the waist to the right or left while shaking the FlexBar challenges the core.

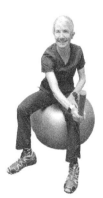

A 2018 article published in the Journal of Physical Therapy Sciences, "Effects of Stabilization Exercise Using Flexi-bar on Functional Disability and Transverse Abdominis Thickness in Patients With Chronic Low Back Pain," evaluated the benefits of adding a Flexbar to core stabilization exercises. People performed 30 minutes of exercise three times per week for six weeks.
https://www.ncbi.nlm.nih.gov/pmc/articles/PMC5857446/
One group performed stability exercises by adding a Flexbar to further challenge proprioception and stabilization. While the control group performed the same exercises without the Flexbar. Adding the Flexbar increased stimulus to the deep spinal stabilizer muscles, producing greater improvement in functional stability and reduced pain levels.

Many people think they need to lift heavy weights to exhaustion to gain strength and endurance, but that is not true. Functional workouts often provide greater benefit to people because they challenge the weakest muscle groups and neuromuscular control systems.

This exercise can be performed standing on the ground, foam, or unstable surface. Sitting on the ball with changing foot position also challenges the core and balance system.

FlexBar Exercises
The TheraBand FlexBar is a great tool for developing arm strength and coordination. Rubber FlexBars come in different widths and stiffness, so you can use them to rehab an injury or to enhance your strength in a key area.

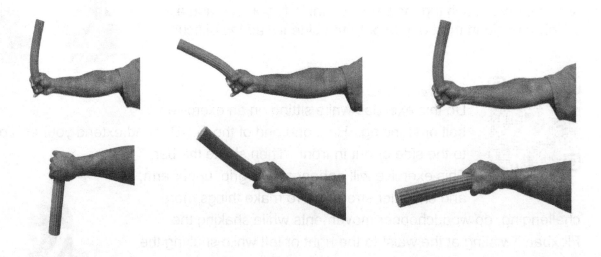

Equipment

Stability exercises are made more difficult when using a few simple and inexpensive pieces of exercise equipment.

Stretch Bands - Simple and effective for increasing hamstring and hip stretching.
https://amzn.to/2rbBPG5

Foam Pads- Are simple foam pads that make all standing exercises slightly more difficulty. Foam challenges the proprioceptive systems by making the surface softer and more difficult to stand on. -https://amzn.to/36CZjEy -

Exercise Balls - Therapeutic exercises balls are used for a variety of lower back and core exercises. This is the best $20 you can spend on your health. Buying, inflating, and using this ball can be tremendous for your lower back and core muscles.
https://amzn.to/34BB5IZ

Kettlebells - Dumbbell weights can be used for the following exercises too. I personally like kettlebells for additional strengthening and stability exercises, along with its ability to use on the exercise balls or foam. A 5, 10, and 20 lbs weights can complete an exercise set and provide many treatment options. https://amzn.to/34BB5IZ

Vibration Plates - These are fantastic at increasing core, back, hip, knee, ankle, and foot strength. We regularly utilize these in the office, and when used at home can enhance your strength and complete your workout room. These will challenge your neuromuscular, strength, and endurance systems more than any other piece of equipment. https://amzn.to/2JPfFA4

Balance and Chronic Back Pain

A person with chronic low back pain also loses balance and stability while standing and walking. For example, the ability to stabilize oneself when standing on one foot decreases with chronic low back pain. As a person's condition continues to deteriorate, the single leg stance stability worsens. The poor balance is a consequence of pain and poor proprioception from the low back facet joints, and weakness and loss of stability from the deep spinal stabilizer muscles.

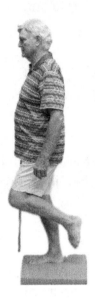

This is not a new concept. A study published in 1998 in the journal *Spine* titled "One-Footed and Externally Disturbed Two-Footed Postural Control in Patients with Chronic Low Back Pain and Healthy Control Subjects: A Controlled Study with Follow Up" evaluated this principle.

The study concluded: "Postural stability is easily disturbed in case of impairment in strength, coordination, or effective coupling of muscles in the lumbar and pelvic area. Patients with chronic low back pain seem to experience impairment in these functions, which should be taken into consideration when back rehabilitation programs are planned."
https://www.ncbi.nlm.nih.gov/pubmed/9794052

Building on the recommendations of the prior study, a 2018 study published in the *Journal of Exercise Rehabilitation*, "Comparison of the Effects of Stability Exercise and Balance Exercise on Muscle Activity in Female Patients with Chronic Low Back Pain," showed that back pain was reduced in both stability and balance exercise groups, through different mechanisms. https://www.ncbi.nlm.nih.gov/pmc/articles/PMC6323339/

A similar finding appeared in a 2018 study published in the *BMC Musculoskeletal Disorder Journal* titled "Postural Awareness and its Relationship to Pain: Validation of an Innovative Instrument Measuring Awareness of Body Posture in Patients with Chronic Pain." The study found that improving posture decreased spinal and shoulder pain.
https://www.ncbi.nlm.nih.gov/pubmed/29625603

For this reason we combine traditional strengthening exercises with stability and balance exercises to reduce back pain and enhance spinal stability.

Watch the Video: Why Most People Have Chronic Lower Back Pain

Foundation Low Back Exercises

<u>Bridging exercises</u>
Start on your back with knees bent and feet shoulder width apart. Slowly raise your waist toward the ceiling, trying to pick your pelvis up toward the ceiling but not extending your back. The idea is to create a straight line from your shoulder through the waist and to the knees. Concentrate on slow and steady movements up and down, keeping the waist level at all times. Avoid swaying or tipping the pelvis during the movement.

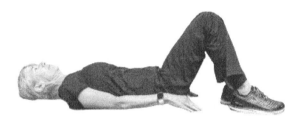 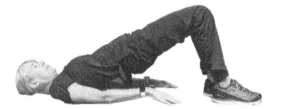

Bridging exercises start with two feet apart and then move to two feet together. Then move to a position with one foot on top of the other and next, on one leg with the lifted knee bent. Finally, the lifted knee is kept straight. The progression is mastering 3 sets of 10 with two feet apart before moving on to two feet together. Then progress to one foot on top of the other for 3 sets of 10 before moving onto single-leg position.

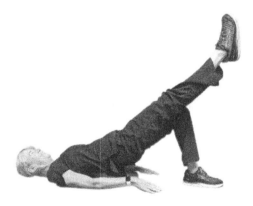

Glute bridge Ball:
The glute bridge builds strength in all of the gluteal muscles: Maximus, Minimus and Medius. The ball makes you unstable and requires more core stabilization and strength. Eyes can be open or closed for increased difficulty.

Roll out on the ball until it is resting under your shoulders, supporting your upper back. As with the plank position, having your feet shoulder width apart makes the exercise easier, whereas keeping the feet and knees together is more challenging. Cross your arms across the chest. Slowly lower your hips to the floor and then raise them back up to a tabletop position. Watch out for any side-to-side movement (usually indicating pelvic instability from weak hip stabilizers). Also, be careful not arch your back, since this can cause lower back strain. Repeat ten times for two-to-three sets.

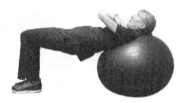 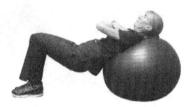

45, 90, 180 Laying on Bench
Laying flat on your stomach, raise your leg while keeping the knee straight. The movement should come from extending your hip and not rolling your pelvis. Perform 10 repetitions with the right leg before 10 repetitions with the left. Next, keeping the knee straight and toes pointed toward the floor, move the foot to the side abducting the hip.
You will feel more muscle activation on the side of your glutes. Once again, perform all 10 repetitions before switching legs.

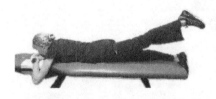

The last part of this exercise is to lift your foot at a 45 degree angle in a linear line. This is the hardest of the three for most people. Only go as far as you can without straining or rotating your femur. Build up to 3 sets of 10 on each leg. To make the exercise harder, go through the movements with a resistance rubber band.

Single leg hip abduction - Toe in / Out/ Straight

Standing on one foot, abduct the raised leg to the side. Concentrate on slow and steady leg movements while maintaining balance. A rubber band can be added around the legs to make it more difficult.

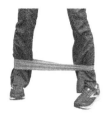

Duck Walks

Side-to-side walks increase lateral hip, knee, and ankle strength. Place a resistance band around your ankles and keep tension on the band throughout the exercise. Initially, move slowly, stepping with the lead leg to the side and even more slowly as you bring the trail leg back toward the middle. Don't lose tension on the band as the trail leg nears the lead leg. There are three positions for duck walk:

1. Toes pointing straight forward the entire time.
2. Toes pointing inward the entire time.
3. Toes point out the entire time.

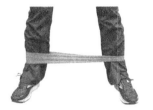 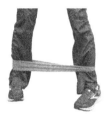 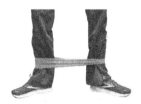

Single leg posterior hip bumps

Stand six inches from a wall on your right leg, with your left held in front. Slowly move backward until you fall into the wall, and then push yourself off the wall with your hips. Once you regain a steady balance on one foot, repeat the exercise. As you improve, move further from the wall.

 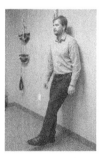

Side hip bumps

Similar to the posterior hip bumps. Standing with your hip facing the wall, fall to the side. Push off the wall with your hips and regain your balance. You will need to start closer to the wall compared to posterior hip bump exercise. Hip bump exercises can be made more difficult by standing on an unstable surface or with your eyes closed.

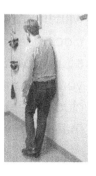

Side step ups
Just like it sounds. Step onto the step sideways. Focus on keeping your waist as level as possible and controlling your torso rock. Step both up and down the steps each direction.

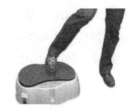

Backward step ups
Practice going up the step backwards. Reverse the exercises stepping down to the ground backwards. Going slowly is much more difficult than moving quickly. Slow movements require you to use more hip stabilizers than when going fast, *so go slow*.

Square Dance
Stand on your right leg with the left held slightly in the air. Keeping all your weight on the right foot, reach the left behind you and tap the ground without supporting any body weight. Then reach the leg forward and tap a point in front of your right leg. Next, reach back and to the left, tapping the ground, then reach forward and to the left. Think of tapping the corners of a square. Repeat 10 times on each leg.

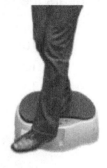

Once you have become comfortable with the square dance exercise, begin crossing behind and in front of your body. When standing on your right leg, your left foot will tap a point behind and to the right of your body. Likewise, when standing on your left leg, tap a point in front and to the left of your body.

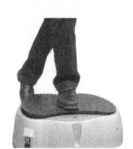

Clock exercise
Think of the face of a watch, not a digital clock. Standing on one foot with the raised foot held behind you, rotate as far as you can counter clockwise. Keeping your hands at your chest and your back straight, squat down as far as you can, maintaining form and balance. Tap your toe onto the ground like the hands of a clock. Slowly rotate clockwise one position and squat again. Work through all the positions of a clock dial that you can, and then repeat going counter clockwise.

Slow walk resistance

With a mild resistance rubber band around your ankles, begin walking in a straight line. Do not move fast. Focus on slow, controlled movements and maintain resistance for most of the movement. The walk can be exaggerated with a swinging leg to the side, or a monster-type walk.

Ball Sitting Rotational Exercises

Sitting on the exercise ball is a great way to engage the core muscles without bending, hinging, or extending. These exercises are great for those individuals who need to increase the coordination between the pelvis, core, back, and scapula. The ball seated exercises are also great for those who have chronic low back pain and just can't seem to get better.

Each of the exercises can be made easier by sitting with the feet wide apart. Moving the feet closer together makes each exercise harder. Raising one foot off the ground makes the exercise even more difficult. As with the standing exercises, closing the eyes makes all of the exercises more difficult and requires the balance system to work together to keep you from falling off the exercise ball. **Be safe.**

Moderate Exercises

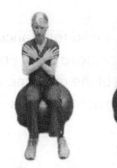 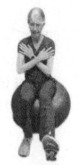

Seated leg-raise
Sit on the ball with your arms crossed. Slowly raise the left leg, lower it and then raise the right leg. Repeat ten times with each leg for a set. Eventually you can add a weight to hold in front of you or to the side for added difficulty.

Abdominal Curl Up
The ball should be positioned to support your lower and middle back. With your arms positioned so that your hands are supporting your head and neck, tighten abdominal muscles and curl up slowly. Return to the original (supine) position. To add challenge, twist while curling, first to the left and then to the right.

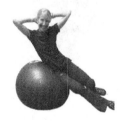

Lateral curl up
Start with your feet on the floor, lying on your side with the ball under your hips. You may want to prop one of your feet against a wall to anchor yourself. Curl up sideways, then lower back down to the starting position. Repeat for a total of ten lifts on each side.

Cross Crawl Ball
Start in a prone position with your hands and feet touching the floor and the ball under your trunk. Slowly lift the left arm and right leg off the floor and extend them so the they are aligned with the body (straight out to the front and back). Lower them back to the starting position and lift the opposite limbs. A set consists of ten lifts on each side.

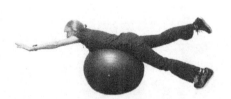

Inner and outer thigh lift
Start out lying on your side, with the ball positioned between the feet and lower legs. Raise both legs up towards the ceiling,

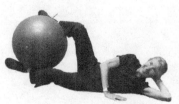

192

keeping them in alignment with your trunk. Repeat for a total of ten lifts, then switch sides (ten more lifts) for one set.

Hamstring curls

Begin by lying prone on the mat, elbows out and head resting on your hands. Grab the ball between your feet and lower legs. Bend the knees and slowly lift the ball towards the ceiling, then lower it back down to the floor. Repeat nine more times for a set.

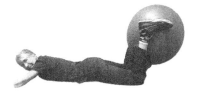

Plank on the ball

For beginners, start with your feet slightly apart and the ball under your chest. Your head, shoulders, back, hips and legs should ideally form a straight line. Raising your hips too high makes the plank easier but less effective, while letting them fall towards the ground can cause lower back pain.

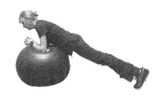

Once you have mastered this position, progress by positioning your forearms on the ball with the elbows slightly apart and hands together. To make the position more difficult, bring your feet together. Then try lifting one leg off the ground.

Plank and roll

Before you attempt this exercise, you should be able to hold the plank position on the ball for 30 seconds. Start out in the plank position on the ball. Roll the ball back and forth under you, keeping your hips and feet stable. Your body should stay in its original position and not move with the ball. Roll forwards and backwards 10-12 times for a set. Fun twist: Move the ball in a circular pattern, clockwise and counter-clockwise.

Push-up

In a prone position, roll out on the ball until it is somewhere between your knees and feet. Think of the ball as a fulcrum: the further it is from the center

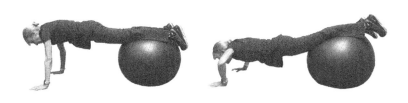

of your body, the more challenging it is to do push-ups. Just as with conventional push-ups, it's important to keep your head, shoulders, back, hips and legs in alignment.

Start with one set of ten and work your way up to two-or-three sets.

Lateral Hip Strength Exercises with Slider & Rubber Band

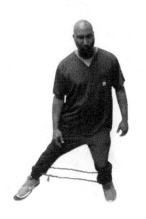

The slider helps to focus on slow and controlled movements and the rubber band adds resistance to build strength and endurance.

Move the foot as if reaching for the numbers on a clock and work all the way around. Turning the foot also subtly changes the exercises as you move through the progression. The exercise can be made more difficult by holding a weight, a stiffer rubber band, or using an elevated platform.

Lunge Step with Sliders

Step down and lunge exercises can progress to using a step and a slider. Start with small step and slider movements and progress to larger movements with improvement. Slide as if touching all the numbers on a clock to develop full hip and pelvic range of motion and strength. The slider helps to slow the movement and enhances the exercise into all directions of movement.

Start with slow and controlled movements and increase the stride with improvement.
The exercise can be made more difficult by using a taller step, adding a weight, or using a rubber band.

Ball wall squat

Start by leaning with your back against the ball, and the ball positioned in the small of your back. Your legs should be straight and feet slightly forward, so that your knees don't move forward of your toes when you squat.

Initially squat a few inches to focus on glute strength and activation. With improvement, squat lower and lower. Eventually your knees form a ninety-degree angle, then return to a standing position. Start with one set of ten and work your way up to two-to-three sets.

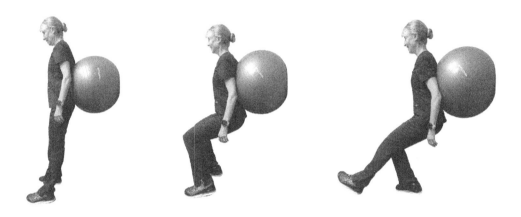

To make this exercise more challenging, hold a medicine ball straight above your head when you squat. Doing so creates a longer lever, requiring you to use more muscles. It will also remind you not to bend forward when you squat, maintaining proper form.

Ball squat (without the wall):
Hold the exercise ball between your hands with your arms straight out in front of you. Slowly squat down, then return to the standing position. Repeat nine more times.

Seated Ball Rotational Twists

Sitting on the ball with feet shoulder width apart, slowly rotate the torso to the left. Pause for a few seconds and then rotate toward the right, pausing at the end range of motion. These exercises can be made more

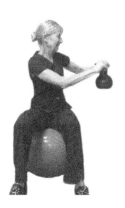

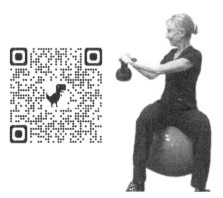

difficult by moving your feet closer together or holding a weight in your hands. Eventually the weight can be held in front of the torso during the movements.

Seated ball chop
A variation of the medicine ball woodchopper exercise, sitting on the ball with hands in front. Reach up and to the right with arms extended, and then reach down to the left. A medicine ball or small weight can be used for added difficulty. Perform this exercises in both directions.

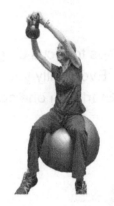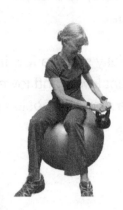

<u>Medicine Ball Woodchopper</u>

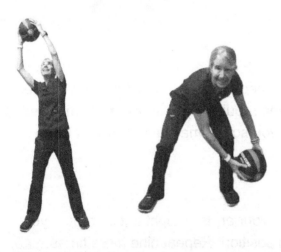

Begin standing with feet shoulder width apart, holding the medicine ball straight out in front of you. Reach up and to the right with your arms extended, then bring the ball down and to the left, bending your knees for a full range-of-motion. Your back should remain straight and flexed slightly forward. Keeping the arms straight, bring the ball up on the left-hand side and fully extend your arms, now swing it down and to the right, bending the knees as you go. Ten "chops" in each direction is one set.

Rear medicine ball raise
Grab the medicine ball behind your back. With your arms straight, lift the ball up towards the ceiling. Repeat for a total of ten lifts in a set.

Moderate Hard Exercises

The foundation of exercises have to be mastered to move onto these exercises. Skipping steps will cost you later.

Single leg ball wall squats
Next, perform single leg squats. Try to move slowly and controlled through the exercise while pausing at the bottom of the squat. Another form of the exercise is to squat and hold the position for 30 seconds before standing.

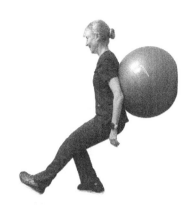

Single leg squats
Standing on one leg with the other knee bent, keep your back straight as you squat downward, until the point where you want to hinge forward. Over time, you will be able to squat lower before hinging. Start squatting on the ground, then add unstable surfaces to increase the challenge.

Split squats

Take a large forward step and keep your legs apart. Keeping your back straight, lower your waist toward the ground. Stop as it becomes too difficult to keep the back straight or maintain balance. Your knees should continue to point forward, and your waist should not rotate or wobble.

These squats are used as a transition to build strength and endurance toward a forward and backward lunge. For added difficulty, place a piece of foam or towel under one leg to make it more unstable.

To focus on the glutes make sure the lower leg of the lead is pointing backwards. When the knee moves forward and the tibia is pointing forward the exercise uses more quads. When the tibia is pointing backwards the glutes can be emphasized.

For a quad dominant person having the tibia pointing backwards is very awkward. Start by only lowering the pelvis a couple inches and focus on using your glutes. With improvement the pelvis can be lowered further to the ground. The same process as with ball wall squats and single leg ball wall squats.

Around the world

Around the world teaches you to stabilize your hips and knees while bending and twisting. Begin by marking three spots on the floor: one directly in front of you, one to the left (about 60-degrees from the front mark), and one to the right (also 60 degrees from the front mark). Stand on one leg and using an exercise ball, bend and reach for the left mark. Touch the ball to the left mark, middle mark and right mark, returning to a standing position between each ball touch.

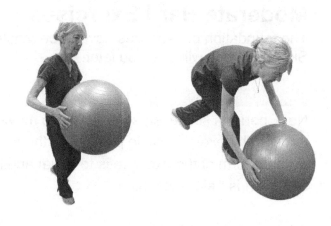

You should touch each mark 3-4 times before switching legs and repeating the exercise. Performing the exercise on both legs constitutes one set.

Hamstring Ball Curl

Laying on your back with two feet on an exercise ball, lift your waist into the air. Next, pull your feet into the ball and roll it toward your waist. The harder you pull into the ball, the more stress will be applied to the hamstring muscles. After you pull the ball as far as you can, extend your legs as you maintain pressure into the ball. The exercise can be performed with two feet or a single leg.

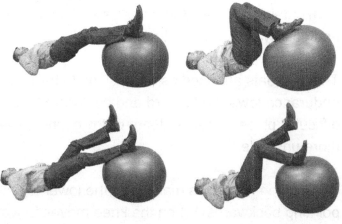

Mountain climber

We do this exercise using the treatment tables, but you can do it at home using your bed (if the mattress is relatively firm) or a table. You can also do it at the gym using a flat weight bench. Begin in the plank position. If you do the plank correctly, your head, shoulders, hips and knees should form a straight line. It's important not to sag in the middle or raise your hips up too high so that you are angled at the waist. Drive one knee towards the table and move it back to the original position, then drive forward with the opposite knee. This exercise is about building power and strength, so move quickly, just as if you were climbing an actual mountain. Drive each knee forward ten times to complete a set.

Mountain climber on exercise ball

Before you attempt the mountain climber, you should feel comfortable performing the mountain climber on a bench or table as well as being able to hold a plank on an exercise ball for 30 seconds. To perform the 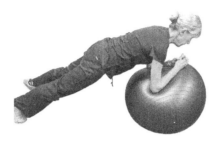 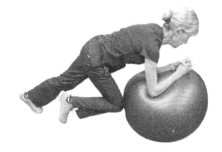 mountain climber, get into the plank position on the ball. Kick one knee forward until it touches the ball, then move it back into place and kick with the other knee. Kick the ball 10 times with each knee for one complete set.

Forward ball tuck

Begin by rolling yourself forward on the exercise ball until the ball is under your feet and your arms are fully extended to the floor. This is similar to the position you would assume for push ups on the exercise ball. Move your knees to your chest: the exercise ball should roll forward under your legs and in the full-tuck position, be close to your hands. Extend your knees and roll the ball back to its original position. Repeat for a total of 10 tucks for a set.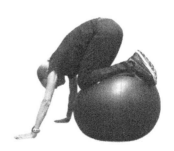

Reverse ball tuck

This is a more challenging exercise for those who have mastered the ball tuck. Sit on an exercise mat and position the exercise ball under your feet. Your knees should be bent to about 90 degrees. Position your arms by your side so your hands are on the floor right next to your hips. Your hands should be slightly angled out from your body. Extend your arms fully so your hips are off the floor. Use your feet to roll the ball away from you until your legs are almost fully extended, then roll the ball backwards towards your hips. Roll the ball back and forth ten times, then lower your hips back slowly to the floor to complete a set.

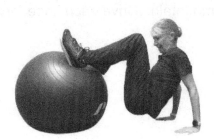 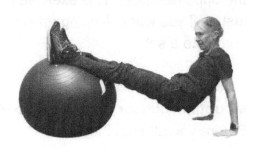

Dips on the ball

This is a fun challenge for anyone who has mastered dips off of an exercise bench. By using an exercise ball, you need to work much harder to stabilize your hips and knees. Start by sitting on the exercise ball with your legs extended slightly out in front of your knees. Position your hands next to your hips with fingers facing forward. Carefully lift, push your hips up off the ball, move forward, and lower your hips towards the floor. Then push your hips up and back onto the ball. Complete 10 dips for a full set.

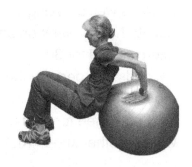

Prone Flies on the Ball

Start in a prone position with the exercise ball under your chest, holding a dumbbell in each hand, and arms lowered to the floor as much as possible. With the arms extended out but slightly curled (see above), raise the weights up until they are slightly above your torso, then lower them back down to the starting position. Repeat a total of 10 times for a set.

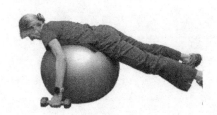 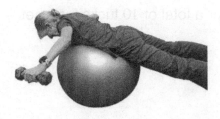

One Arm Row

Do this exercise from a quadruped position on a yoga mat, with one foot on the ground and one knee bent on a weight bench. Or for a greater challenge, start in the plank position. When doing rows, be sure to keep your elbow close to the body. Grab a dumbbell and begin the exercise with your arm fully extended. It can be straight down if you are on a bench. If you are starting in a quadruped position, you may need to extend the arm slightly forward. Starting from the plank position, the arm will be extended down with the weight on the ground.

Slowly bring the weight up towards your waist keeping the elbow bent and close to the torso. Then lower the weight down to the starting position and repeat 10 times for a set. Repeat a set of 10 using the opposite arm.

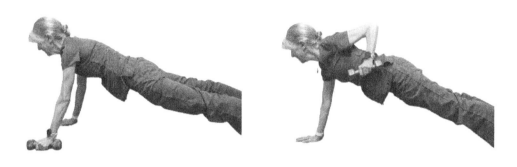

Bear Crawl & Crab Walk: These exercises remind many of highschool P.E. and sports. These exercises are excellent at stabilizing the scapula. The exercises can be performed holding the positions or moving across the floor. At first we recommend holding the position to fatigue for 3-5 reps. With improvement then start walking across the floor.

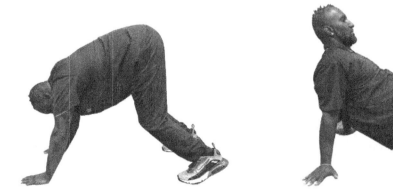

Wall Slides

Standing and facing a wall place your arms at 90 degrees with the forearms on the wall. Glide the forearms straight up the wall as far as comfortable. A variation is to angle the arms up the wall as if you are trying to make a "Y" with your arms.

A rubber band can be placed between the forearms for added resistance.

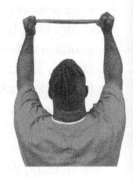

Wall Angels

With your back against the wall, place your arms and elbow at 90 degrees against the wall. Keep the wrist, elbows, scapula, and pelvis against the wall and raise your arms toward the ceiling. Glide the arms against the wall until you feel a strong stretch or a part of your body

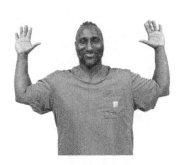
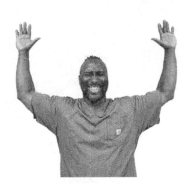

starts to lift off the wall. With improvement your arms will be able to glide higher up the wall. A resistance band can also be utilized for added difficulty.

Y-T-W-L

A great stretch for the chest, shoulders, and upper back. Similar to performing the motions to the song YMCA, instead you will be performing YTWL. Repeat 3 times. The Y-T-W-L can be performed as a stretch. It can also incorporate bands and small weights. It can be performed standing, sitting on a ball, or laying prone on bench.

Y - Make a big Y with your arms with the elbows straight, and then pull the arms backwards until you feel a comfortable stretch. Hold for 10 seconds.

Performing the **Y-T-W-L** with resistance exercise bands. Slow and smooth, concentration on keeping the scapula low. These are great exercises to focus on eccentric movements.

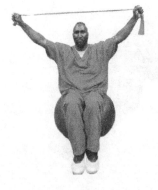
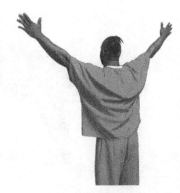

T - Lower your arms and form a T, once again pulling the arms backwards for a comfortable 10 second stretch.

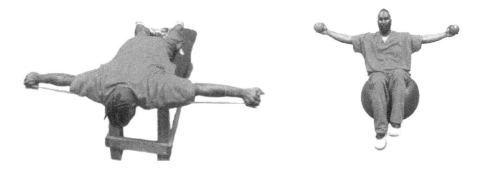

W - From the T position bend your elbows with them lowering toward the ground, form a W with your arms.

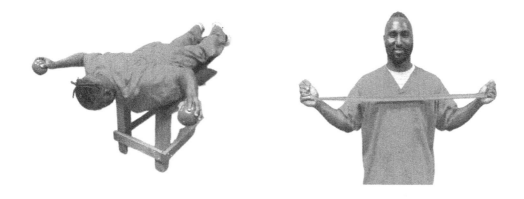

L - From the W position, lower your hands until a 90 degree bend occurs at the elbow. The elbow should be touching the torso. Stretch the hands backwards for 10 seconds.

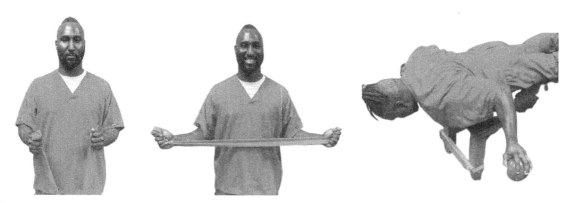

Performing the **Y-T-W-L** with resistance exercise bands. Slow and smooth, concentration on keeping the scapula low. These are great exercises to focus on eccentric movements.

FlexBar Shake

Do this exercise while sitting on an exercise ball or standing. Progress from a two foot stance to tandem or single leg.

Hold one end of the FlexBar and extend your arm out to the side or out in front. Then shake the bar. This exercise will enhance your grip, upper arm, and shoulder strength. To make things more challenging, do woodchopper movements while shaking the Flexbar. Twisting at the waist to the right or left while shaking the FlexBar challenges the core.

A 2018 article published in the Journal of Physical Therapy Sciences, "Effects of Stabilization Exercise Using Flexi-bar on Functional Disability and Transverse Abdominis Thickness in Patients With Chronic Low Back Pain," evaluated the benefits of adding a Flexbar to core stabilization exercises. People performed 30 minutes of exercise three times per week for six weeks.
https://www.ncbi.nlm.nih.gov/pmc/articles/PMC5857446/

One group performed stability exercises by adding a Flexbar to further challenge proprioception and stabilization. While the control group performed the same exercises without the Flexbar. Adding the Flexbar increased stimulus to the deep spinal stabilizer muscles, producing greater improvement in functional stability and reduced pain levels.

Flexbar provides a similar stimulus to the upper extremity that standing on a vibration plate does for the lower extremity.

Many people think they need to lift heavy weights to exhaustion to gain strength and endurance, but that is not true. Functional workouts often provide greater benefit to people because they challenge the weakest muscle groups and neuromuscular control systems.

Anterior Plank

Basic Plank: You can perform a plank using a wall (easiest), raised bench, on a floor mat (more challenging), or on an exercise ball (even more challenging). The easiest progression is starting from your knees and moving to your toes with progress. Watch the progression

Watch the full anterior plank progression from knees to progressing to toes.

Side planks and reverse planks are variations on the basic prone plank that work your core muscles in different ways and challenge the scapular stabilizers to control forces at the shoulder joints.

The important thing to remember here is: Start low and go slow. Begin with the level of difficulty you can master with proper form. Here are a few things to keep in mind:

1. Keep the shoulders down and back. The tendency is to hunch the shoulders when performing a plank, especially if your core muscles aren't quite up to the task. This is a good way to develop upper back pain. As a trainer, I will occasionally place a dowel rod on the person's back to emphasize the line I would like to see from the head to the feet.
2. Keep your butt in line with the rest of your body. Raising it up makes the plank easier to hold, but it won't give you the benefits (abdominal strengthening) of doing the exercise correctly.
3. Don't let your middle sag. This will likely result in lower back pain.
4. Don't forget to breathe. The body needs oxygen, especially when performing challenging exercises.
5. Only hold the position as long as you can with proper form. If you feel the form starting to fall apart, take a rest. You will get more benefit from multiple shorter reps than a one-minute plank during which you struggle to keep your belly off the floor.

When transitioning to the exercise ball, you might want to start by having somebody spot you (hold the ball until you find your balance). An alternative is to position the ball against a wall or in a corner to add some stability. Lay on your stomach with your forearms underneath your chest. With your tip toes firmly on the ground, lift your waist and body off the ground. Keep your back straight as you create a straight line from your shoulders through the waist, knees and ankles. The tendency is to drop the pelvis or lift the butt in the air as you get tired. Hold the position to fatigue at first, then build up to 3 sets of 2 minutes.

Anterior plank exercises can be performed on your forearms or hands with elbows straight, like the top of a push up position. Moving the hands closer together makes the exercise harder, as does moving the feet closer together. Eventually you can perform a plank on one foot or hand. You can also place an exercise ball or BOSU ball under your hands or toes for added difficulty.

Lateral planks
Start by laying on your right side with your forearm perpendicular to your torso. Lift your waist off the ground while keeping the side of your right foot on the ground. Your left foot will be on top of the right. Focus on keeping your body perpendicular to the ground, and not rocking forward or bending at the waist.

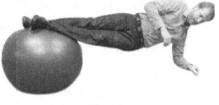

Start by holding the position to fatigue and then switching to the left side. Build up to three sets of 1 minute on each side.

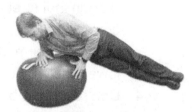

Once again, the exercise can be made more difficult by placing an unstable surface under the hands or feet. Or add a weight to the free hand.

Mike Showing OFF - Vibration & Ball - Plank & Push Up

Lots of ways to challenge yourself, especially with unstable surfaces. If one is good, then two must be better.

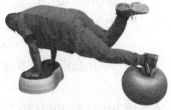

Place your hands on a vibration unit and feet on the ball. Planks, pushups, mountain climbers, and more.

External shoulder rotation

Hold one end of the TheraBand in your hand. Your elbow should be bent, and your hand will be at your body's midsection. Keeping the elbow bent, rotate the band outward. Bring it back to the starting position and repeat 10 times for a set.

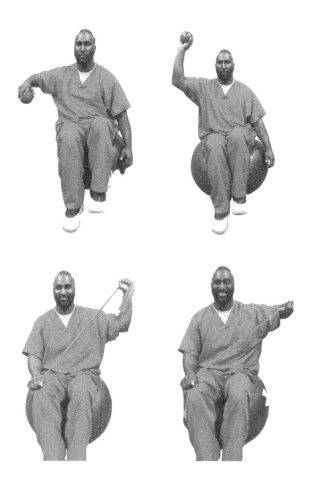

Internal rotation

This is the opposite of the external rotation exercise. Start with the hand rotated away from the body and rotate it inward towards your midline.

Advanced Exercises

Many of the beginner and intermediate exercises can be made more difficult by adding an unstable surface. You can also hold a 5-10-pound weight during the exercises to further challenge the stabilizer muscles.

Vibration platforms make any of the standing exercises harder by knocking you continually off balance. The body has to work harder to maintain balance along with moving through the activity. At our office, we slowly incorporate most standing and squatting exercises onto the vibration plate. Most people are surprised how much harder the exercises become on the vibration plate.

BOSU & vibration single leg stance
Perform single leg stance exercises on the vibration plate. Maintaining balance on one leg while squatting is significantly harder on unstable surfaces. Start with standing on the rubber portion of the BOSU before turning it upside down. Then transition to squatting on the vibration plate.

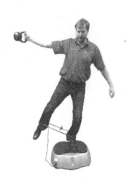

Rotational movements on ball or vibration plate
Standing with either two feet or one foot, squat downward while maintaining an erect posture; no hinging at the low back. With your hands in front of you, rotate to one side and then the other side. Once you get the hang of it, add a weight to your hands. The further you can hold the weight from your body, the harder the exercise becomes, especially on one foot.

Medicine ball wall squat
In a knees-bent, squat position, push your back against the wall. Hold a medicine ball in your hands, With- your arms straight, raise the medicine ball up so it is in front of your chest. Hold the position for thirty seconds, working your way up to two sixty-second holds.

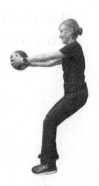

Jumping onto unstable surfaces

Landing on a variety of unstable surfaces further challenges the body's proprioceptive system. Jumping from and onto foam, wobble boards, rocker boards, vibration plates, and elevated surfaces is the next step in the progression. Click to read and see more examples.

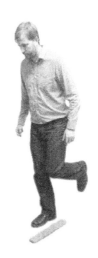

Square jumps

Visualize a box six inches by six inches on the ground. With two feet together, jump from corner to corner. Start going clockwise and then switch to a counter clockwise direction. If you are stable and under control, begin jumping diagonally across the box. Over time, the box can get bigger and bigger. Transition from two-foot jumps to single leg.

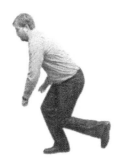 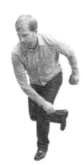

Skier jumps

Standing on your right leg, jump laterally to your left and land on your left leg only. After establishing your balance, laterally jump to the right. Start jumping slowly and establish your balance before jumping the other direction. With improvement, jump further and faster.

Single leg jumps onto vibration plate

Standing on your right leg, jump forward onto the vibration plate. Land and regain your balance before jumping forward off the vibration plate and then quickly jumping forward again. After improving on the forward jumps, stand on the right side of the plate on jump laterally to your left, landing on the plate. Once again, regain full control before jumping laterally off the plate and onto the ground, quickly jumping to the left upon impact. Repeat the exercise jumping to the right. Once comfortable, you can attempt jumping backwards onto the plate and off

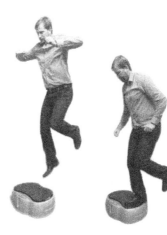

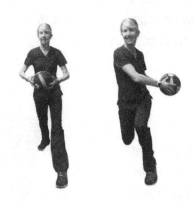

Lunge with Medicine Ball Twist
Stand with your feet slightly apart, holding the medicine ball in front of you. Lunge forward with the left leg, while swinging the medicine ball to the right. Return to the standing position while moving the ball back to midline. Repeat for a total of ten lunges and twists on each side.

A reverse lunge is also a great exercise for hip and lower extremity strength. The exercise is performed with a step backwards and then squat. Lunges can focus on quadriceps or glute strength depending how they are performed.

Russian twist
Start in a supine position (lying on your back) with your knees bent and feet on the floor. Grab the medicine ball between your hands and lift your feet off the floor. Curl up and twist to one side, then come back to neutral and twist to the other side. Twisting to each side ten times is a set.

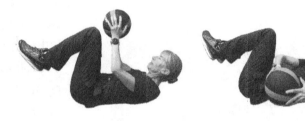

Medicine ball pull-over
Roll the ball out so you are supine with the exercise ball supporting your upper back. Hold the medicine ball between your hands and extend your arms straight up so the ball is above your chest. Keeping the arms straight, extend the ball so it is slightly in back of your head. Then move the ball back to the starting position keeping the arms straight. Repeat nine more times for a set.

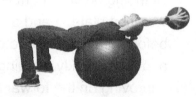

Medicine ball "skull crusher"

Do this exercise with a spotter, since it involves lowering the medicine ball over your head. Roll out on the exercise ball supine until it is supporting your upper back. Holding the medicine ball between your hands, extend your arms so the ball is straight above your chest. Now bend your elbows and lower the

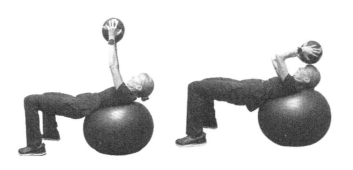

ball towards your forehead. Straighten your arms until the ball is back at the starting position above your chest. Repeat nine more times for a set.

Medicine ball reverse crunch

Lie supine on the mat, with your knees bent and feet on the mat. Grab the medicine ball between your knees and bring your knees up so that your thighs are at a 90-degree angle to your chest. Now bring the ball as close to your chest,

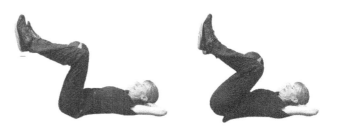

holding it between your knees as possible. Move back to the overhead (90-degree angle) position and repeat an additional nine times for one set.

Rows and Flies on a Mat or Bench

You can do rows or flies on a yoga mat, a weight bench, or while standing. Many of the previous standing exercises above can be performed on unstable surfaces. Progress from the ground to a foam balance pad to BOSU. With improvement you could try performing these exercises on a vibration plate. Each of these unstable surfaces can be made harder by closing one or both eyes. Try it when you are ready, but be safe.

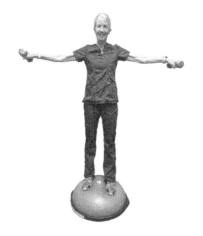 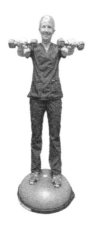 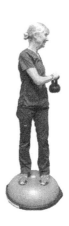

Time For Some Humility Exercises

Reverse plank
Lie supine on the mat with your legs together and straight out in front of you. Bring your forearms and elbows to your side, and slowly raise your torso and hips off the ground so that your torso and legs form a straight line from the shoulders to the knees. Hold this position for 30-to-60 seconds. For a more challenging exercise, raise one leg off the floor while in the plank position.

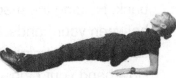

Lower back strengthener
Lie face down on the mat, with your arms straight and hands clasped behind you. Slowly raise your chest and shoulders off the floor and arch your back. Hold for a count of three and return to the starting position. Repeat nine more times for a set.

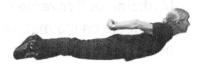

Teaser
Start out in the supine position on the mat. Raise your head and shoulders off the mat and grab your knees. Extend your arms and legs out in a V-position. Bring your arms forward and hold them out straight in front of you so that they touch your legs. Raise and lower the legs three-to-five times, touching your hands to your legs each time.

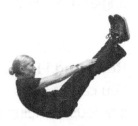

Push-up and dips on the exercise ball
You have already learned how to do push-ups on the ball in the basics section. To do a dip on the ball, start by sitting on the exercise ball with your hands near your hips, palms down and fingers facing forward. Slowly lift yourself up off the ball and lower your butt down towards the ground in front of it. Your knees should remain bent with your feet on the floor. Now using your arms (don't cheat with your legs), raise yourself back up onto the ball in the seated starting position.

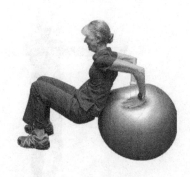

To make this exercise challenging, do a cut-down alternating push ups and dips on the ball.

Forward and reverse tuck

To perform the forward tuck. Start in a prone position and roll out on the exercise ball until the ball is underneath your lower legs, slightly ahead of your feet. Your body should be straight, with your head, shoulders, torso and legs in alignment. Now bend your knees and roll the ball towards your waist until you are in a tuck position. Slowly roll the ball back out to the starting position.

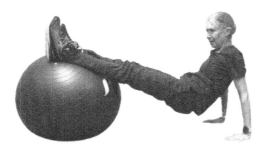 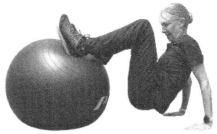

The reverse tuck works opposing muscle groups. Begin by sitting on the ground with your legs straight out in front and feet resting slightly apart on the ball. Your hands should be next to your hips, palms down and fingers either to the sides or facing front. Raise your butt off the ground and slowly roll the ball towards you, bending your knees as you go. Return the ball to the starting position.

This superset is a cutdown, alternating forward and reverse tucks.

As always, be reasonable. Make progress with the exercises. Prove you can and then do a little more.

Mountain climber and glute bridge

You will have learned about the glute bridge in the basics section.

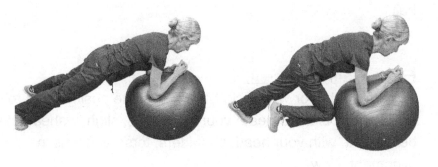

The mountain climber on an exercise ball is a variation on the ball plank. Once in the plank position, kick one knee towards the ball, then move it back to the plank position and kick the other knee forward. You should move your legs quickly, similar to running up a hill.

Alternate the mountain climber and glute bridge for a superset that works the pelvis, abdominal and leg muscles.

Plank with leg extension; medicine ball raise and touch

We mentioned the plank with leg extension briefly in the basics section. From the plank-on-ball position, slowly raise one leg behind you, keeping the leg straight, and then lower it back to the starting position. Alternate leg raises.

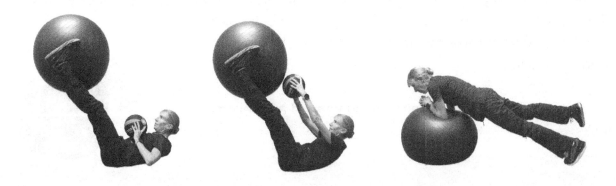

To perform the medicine ball raise and touch, start out supine on the mat. Grab the exercise ball between your feet and lower legs and raise it straight up, so that your legs (and the ball) are at a ninety-degree angle to the floor. Grab the medicine ball between your hands and curl up so the head and shoulders are off the floor. Touch the medicine ball to the exercise ball, bring it back down to the starting position and repeat.

Pommel Horse

This exercise is incredible at challenging the lower scapular stabilizers. With the hands at your side, lift the torso off the ground. Hold the position until fatigue and rest. Repeat several times. At first position the feet so they are supporting some of the body weight, and with strength move the feet further from your body. A variation is to place a block or small exercise ball under the feet with the legs extended.

A few individuals can lift their feet off the ground while supporting their weight, like a gymnast on the pommel horse. Mike was able to hold his torso and feet off the ground with the vibration plate running, which was impressive. It requires significant scapular, shoulder, and core strength. It is a very difficult exercise goal and why we listed it last on the exercise sheet. Good luck!

Kettlebells

Kettlebells can be a great tool for enhancing strength, endurance, and power. They can be used for slow concentric or eccentric contractions, and also dynamic loads. Start slow. People have a tendency to hurt themselves the first few times they use kettlebells. They can be used as standard weight and then progress to swinging exercises. Learn from someone who knows what they are doing, not a clip from YouTube.

Kneeling on the Ball

Many of the same exercises can be performed kneeling on the ball. Just as sitting on the ball with two feet together or single leg made the exercise harder, activating the core to maintain balance.

Kneeling on the ball is a step harder, making the lower body work with the pelvis, core, back, scapula, and upper extremity to maintain balance.

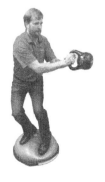 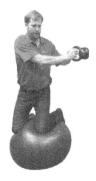 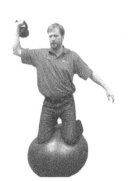 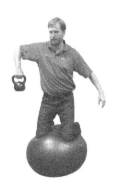

Books by Carson Robertson DC

Low Back Treatment Guide

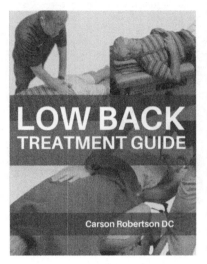

This book offers multiple conservative approaches to managing back pain at home and in the office. It provides several treatment options and strategies to improve your quality of life and eliminate debilitating back pain through a combination of non-invasive treatments and corrective exercise. After reading this book, you'll have the tools to take a more educated look in the mirror; to discover postural problems, dysfunctional movements, and daily habits that may be contributing to your condition. It would be misleading to promise that this book can "cure" your low back pain. What this book can do is help you manage your pain, improve your quality of life, and enjoy your recreational activities. You'll learn to be a better advocate for your own body, leading to a healthier and happier life.

Ultimate Knee Guide For Getting Rid of Pain & Avoiding Surgery: For Those with Grey Hair, Lots of Experience, & Some Wisdom

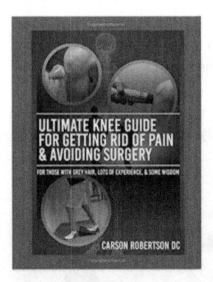

A guide to all conservative and medical treatments available to reduce your knee pain. A variety of knee conditions, home therapies, home products, and exercises are explained to educate and inform you of options available. Most people can successfully avoid knee surgery if they follow the correct treatments and exercise program. Unfortunately most people do not get the right treatments or recommendations, which leads them down the path to surgery. Have you talked to providers who are experts at knee rehabilitation? How do you know you are getting the best advice for your specific condition and where do you go to learn and educate yourself? Most cases of chronic knee pain are a slow development of increasing knee pain over time with subtle loss of function; and can be improved with the right therapy and treatments. Too many people make the mistake of having surgery first, and then going for rehabilitation. Maybe they should go for great rehab first and then surgery if absolutely needed.

Plantar Fasciitis Treatment Guide

People with plantar fasciitis become frustrated with the lack of clear answers, fluctuating foot pain, and various opinions. This complete guide reviews causes of plantar fasciitis, home therapies, home products, conservative treatments, medical treatments, alternative treatments, and provides effective exercises.

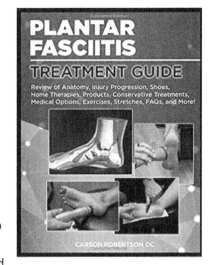

The book clearly explains and educates you on available options. Learn about plantar fasciitis, possible treatments, and home solutions in one book from someone who treats it every day. When do you ice vs heat? When should you consider orthotics or cortisone injections? Is a night splint worth the sleep loss? How big of a role do bone spurs play in heel pain? What are the most effective treatments for breaking up scar tissue and causing proper tissue healing? Most people will require a few different treatments to resolve their foot pain, but which ones provide the greatest benefit?

Elbow Pain Treatment Guide: Elbow Injuries & Treatments - Adults & Seniors

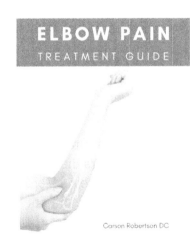

Most adult elbow injuries are the result of overuse and dysfunctional movement patterns. Although this book addresses both acute and chronic injuries, it focuses on the latter due to their high prevalence.

This book focuses on conservative therapies that can be performed at home or in the office for several elbow injuries. Because most elbow injuries don't occur in isolation, this book addresses these injuries within the larger framework of the upper extremity, movement patterns, past injuries, compensation patterns, and chronic repetitive injuries.

Most musculoskeletal injuries can be successfully treated or at worst case managed with a combination of physiotherapy and corrective exercise, especially treatments that focus on muscles, tendons, and ligaments.

Improve Your Game and Reduce Injuries: Simple Home Exercises & Stretches To Improve Your Golf Swing and Stay Pain Free

Golf doesn't pose some of the injury risks that high impact sports such as running or basketball do, playing the game with bad form can lead to injury. Although improper golf mechanics may not cause injuries in the short term, they most likely will catch up with the person at some point and possibly sideline him or her.

The purpose of this book is to connect the dots: to explain some of the differences between proper and improper golf mechanics, how improper movements are leading to injury, and most importantly, what can be done to fix them.

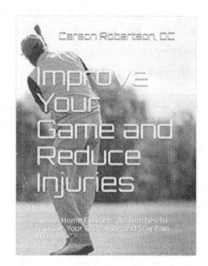

Hand & Wrist Treatment Guide For Adults

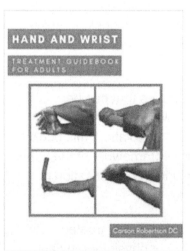

This book offers multiple conservative treatment approaches to improving and managing hand and wrist pain at home and in the office. Many patients require a combination of treatments to decrease pain and enhance tissue repair. The treatment guide provides several treatment options and strategies to eliminate your pain and get you back to your activities quickly.

This hand and wrist book provides multiple treatment strategies for those who want to do it on their own. It also covers the most effective office treatments, for those who need more help. More importantly, it describes treatment options for those who are not improving with basic office therapy. There are more options available than you think.

Upper Extremity Exercises for Adults & Seniors

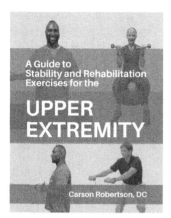

A variety of exercises to increase strength, flexibility, and range of motion for the upper extremity. It includes a variety of rehabilitation and strengthening exercises for adults and seniors to safely return from injury and enhance their functional abilities. This guide includes exercises that incorporate core and scapular strength with shoulder stabilization exercises to give adults an efficient set of progressive exercises to return from injury. It should be obvious an older body shouldn't be given the same exercises as the 20-year-old baseball player, so these exercises combine progressive stabilization exercises with functional abilities that adults can utilize to stay pain free and enjoy their daily activities. It includes the simpletest exercises to perform with an injury and ends with much harder exercises for the most motivated adults.

Stretch Series For Adults - With Average to Poor Flexibility

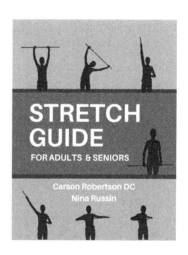

Stretching can be confusing for many, especially if their introduction was in high school gym class. Stretching should be comfortable, *not* painful. There are hundreds of ways to stretch the body, but the best stretches are the ones a person can do safely, comfortably, and consistently. The stretches you performed in high school are probably not feasible now, so this book combines multiple simple stretches for every region of the body. Be safe, consistent, and make progress to enhance your overall flexibility without causing injury.

Lower Extremity Exercises for Adults & Seniors

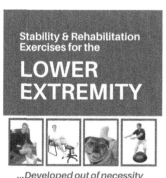

This exercise guide combines very simple to more advanced exercises for adults and those with gray hair. It includes modifications and stepping stone exercises starting from the most limited ability to more advanced. Ever gone to therapy and noticed you were given the exact same exercises as the teenager? Are those really the best exercises for an older body with some wear and tear on it? Functional abilities and goals are very different for those with a little gray hair, and this guide provides several options for accomplishing those functional goals with multiple variations of classic therapy exercises.

Core Exercises for Adults & Seniors

Quality of life and maintaining pain-free activities often involves working on the core and low back muscles. Many of the social media exercises seem too difficult or foreign for adults with gray hair to even attempt. This guide includes progressive stability and core exercises for those who want to be challenged.

The most effective strength training programs are those that require a minimal investment in equipment, and can be done anywhere. An exercise ball and a light weight is all you need.

The Swiss ball provides stimulus to the core muscles because it is inherently unstable. Basically, anything you can do on a weight bench can also be done on an exercise ball be it a bench press, military press, bicep curl, fly or row. The biggest difference between the bench and the ball is that the weight bench allows a person to isolate various parts of the body, whereas the ball, due to its instability, involves the entire body in every exercise. Because of this, you will want to begin with lighter weights, or in some cases, no weights at all.

Shoulder Pain Treatment Guide for Adults & Seniors

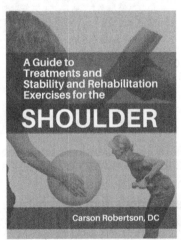

The advantage of a highly mobile shoulder joint is that it gives incredible range of motion and function. The disadvantage is that mobility comes at a cost of less structural protection, leading to increased risk of injury.

The purpose of this book is to explain where your pain came from and the best ways to resolve it at home and in the office. Common shoulder injuries include damage to the rotator cuff muscles (particularly the supraspinatus), impingement, labral tears, frozen shoulder and tendonitis or tendonosis, nerve entrapments, SICK Scapula, upper cross syndrome, thoracic outlet syndrome, and more.

Home and office treatment options are included to enhance your recovery. A variety of exercises are shown from the most basic to advanced. We have included many more than the basics to give you options to strengthen your shoulder and avoid future injuries.

Balance Exercises for Seniors

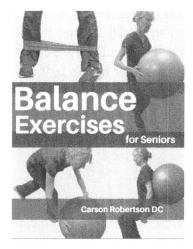

Most people do not notice their balance is slowly deteriorating over years because they never check it. Fortunately your balance can be improved by challenging yourself through a variety of standing and sitting on the ball exercises. This book contains simple balance and stability exercises for those getting started. The ball series starts with sitting on the ball to slowly build core and back stability safely. It progresses to exercises that slowly challenge people at their own pace.

The secret is to "challenge but not overwhelm." In the beginning simple exercises can improve your balance and decrease fall risks. For long term improvement, you need to teach the brain to listen to the lower extremity joints receptors and strengthen the stabilizer muscles.

Ball Exercises - Balance & Stability

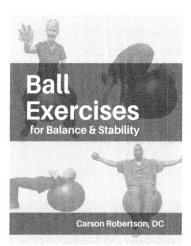

An exercise ball can be an entire workout and most people have never tried more than a few exercises on it. This book contains a variety of exercises for the entire body. It includes simple balance and stability exercises for those getting started. It contains a variety of exercises for the low back and core starting with basic exercises that progress to challenging push ups, planks, and mountain climbers. The series includes a variety of exercises sitting on the ball to slowly build core and back stability safely.

This book provides options on rehab exercises for a shoulder, elbow, or wrist. An exercise ball, bands, and a few weights produces a gym's worth of exercises to perform at home to safely get stronger and avoid injuries.

Max Goes to Sedona: Adventures of Max, Frances, & Lola

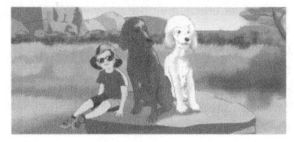

Max goes on a family vacation to Sedona, Arizona. He has a great weekend exploring trails with his best friends, Frances and Lola. The trio finds interesting wildlife as they hike the red dirt trails. They hang out at the pool and visit their first vineyard for Mom's birthday. This is the first of many adventures where Max explores his world with Frances and Lola by his side. He brings his parents along, too, for transportation.

Max Goes to the Zoo: Adventures of Max Frances, & Lola

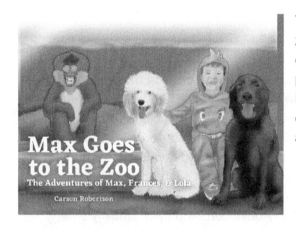

Three-year-old Max tells the story of his trip to the zoo with his best friends, Frances & Lola. He describes the adventure through his eyes, also pointing out what he likes about each animal. Roaring lions, lazy sloths, hungry giraffes, stinky camels, and rattling snakes are just a few stops along the way.

Max Gets Ready for Halloween: Adventures of Max, Frances, & Lola

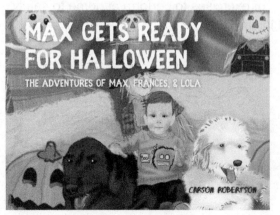

Three-year-old Max tells the story of his Halloweens with his best friends, Frances & Lola. Through his eyes he describes past Halloween costumes & activities. Max loves his family's tradition of going to Mother Nature's Farm to feed the animals, take a hayride, and pick out his pumpkins. Of course, Max also loves his matching costumes with Frances & Lola. Mom always has a theme.

Made in the USA
Monee, IL
20 September 2024